Current themes in rheumatology care

Papers based on an Interfaces in Medicine Conference organised by the Royal College of Physicians, London

Edited by
Ian Lewin MD FRCP
Consultant Physician, North Devon District Hospital Barnstaple, Devon
and
Carol A Seymour PhD FRCP
Professor of Clinical Biochemistry and Metabolism St George's Hospital Medical School, London

1993

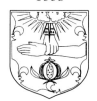

ROYAL COLLEGE OF PHYSICIANS OF LONDON

Acknowledgements

The Royal College of Physicians is grateful to the Arthritis and Rheumatism Council for a generous grant towards the publication of this book.

Royal College of Physicians
11 St Andrews Place, London NW1 4LE

© 1993 Royal College of Physicians of London
ISBN 1 873240 70 8

Typeset by Oxprint Ltd, Aristotle Lane, Oxford OX2 6TR
Printed by The Lavenham Press, Sudbury, Suffolk CO10 9RN.

Contributors

M Anne Chamberlain BSc FRCP *Professor of Rheumatological Rehabilitation, Rheumatology and Rehabilitation Research Unit, University of Leeds Medical School, Leeds LS2 9NZ.*

Peter J Charles FIMLS *Senior Scientific Officer, Department of Rheumatology, Charing Cross Hospital and Division of Clinical Immunology, Kennedy Institute of Rheumatology, London W6 7DW.*

Anthony K Clarke FRCP *Consultant in Rheumatology and Rehabilitation, Royal National Hospital for Rheumatic Diseases, Bath BA1 1RL.*

Colin P Crosby MA MBBS *Sports Medicine Director, Department of Exercise and Sports Medicine, The Garden Hospital, Hendon, London NW4 1RX.*

D John Dickson MBChB MRCGP FRCP(**Glasgow**) *Primary Care Rheumatology Society, 55 South Parade, Northallerton, North Yorkshire DL7 8SL.*

Paul Dieppe BSc MD FRCP *ARC Professor of Rheumatology, Rheumatology Unit, Bristol Royal Infirmary, Bristol BS2 8HW.*

Brian L Hazleman MA FRCP *Consultant Rheumatologist; Director of Rheumatology Research Unit, Addenbrooke's Hospital, Cambridge CB2 2QQ.*

Malcolm IV Jayson MD FRCP *Professor of Rheumatology, Rheumatic Diseases Centre, University of Manchester, Hope Hospital, Salford M6 8HD.*

RN Maini BA FRCP *Professor and Head of Department of Rheumatology, Charing Cross Hospital; Director, The Kennedy Institute of Rheumatology, London W6 7DW.*

J Thomas Scott MD FRCP *Consultant Rheumatologist, Charing Cross Hospital, London W6 8RF.*

Michael L Snaith MD FRCP *ARC Senior Lecturer in Rheumatology, Sheffield Centre for Rheumatic Diseases, Sheffield S11 9EL.*

Patricia Woo PhD FRCP *Head of Section of Molecular Rheumatology and Paediatric Rheumatology Unit, Clinical Research Centre, Northwick Park Hospital, Harrow HA1 3UJ.*

Adam Young MB BChir FRCP *Consultant Rheumatologist, St Albans City Hospital, St Albans, Herts AL3 5PN.*

Editors' introduction

The annual 'Interfaces in Medicine' conferences at the Royal College of Physicians, which were devised by the Standing Committee of Members of the College, provide a forum where general practitioners and physicians can share expertise. Such meetings have become especially welcome during these times of rapid development in healthcare. If met positively, the challenges of changing roles can serve as an opportunity to achieve further excellence in the provision of medical care. Informed and vigorous discussion helps to point the best way forward and this has occurred at the previous conferences in the series which have dealt with cardiovascular disease, asthma and diabetes. 'Current themes in rheumatology care' is based on the fourth of these 'Interfaces' conferences and we are indebted to Dr Matthew Helbert for his assistance with such a comprehensive programme.

This volume opens with an overview of osteoarthritis by Paul Dieppe who also emphasises a principle underpinning all rheumatology, that successful treatment depends upon careful attention to detail. Tom Scott then covers the physiology of hyperuricaemia, defining who should be investigated in depth and clarifying the management of asymptomatic hyperuricaemia as well as reviewing treatment for acute and chronic gout. Brian Hazleman, in the chapter on polymyalgia rheumatica and giant cell arteritis, indicates when temporal artery biopsy can be avoided and describes safe and practical strategies for starting and reducing steroid treatment. Patricia Woo then illustrates some of the more common rheumatic problems of childhood before describing the more serious juvenile chronic arthritides and some of the rarer connective tissue disorders.

Chronic back pain is a common problem and in some patients is intractable. In Chapter 5, Malcolm Jayson describes a role for vascular damage, fibrosis and sympathetic dysfunction in this condition. Increasing understanding of these mechanisms of disease stimulates and allows new approaches to prevention and treatment of chronic back pain.

In a society which increasingly is persuaded towards a healthy lifestyle, there is surprisingly little formal provision for injuries resulting from exercise. In Chapter 6, Colin Crosby describes patterns of sports injuries, ways of preventing them and the setting up of local clinics to deal with them.

John Dickson, in Chapter 7, describes how primary care rheumatology aims to provide quality care at a local level and how it should be cost-effective by identifying accurately the small number of patients who need hospital-based treatment. Using rheumatoid arthritis as an example, he describes the process of diagnosis and assessment, liaison with the hospital specialist and the codes of practice for using second line drug therapy. Contracts between purchasers and providers, as they become more specific, must be made to work to the advantage of the patient, for example by enhancing domiciliary services and hastening access to orthopaedic surgery.

The increasing involvement of primary care, even in complex problems, is argued further by Michael Snaith who describes the presentation and management of systemic lupus erythematosus. He proposes a model of care such that, in a large group practice, one partner might wish to pursue a special interest in the rheumatic diseases, liaising closely with his hospital counterpart and handling such relatively uncommon cases as SLE with greater confidence. Current methods of investigating SLE reveal the major advances in laboratory medicine and in Chapter 9, Peter Charles and Tiny Maini describe how autoantibodies are used in the diagnosis and prognosis of rheumatic diseases.

The last three chapters in this book focus on various other aspects of treatment for the rheumatic diseases. Adam Young balances the risks and benefits of nonsteroidal anti-inflammatory drugs and recommends guidelines for safe prescribing. Anthony Clarke then gives a systematic guide to the injection of joints and periarticular tissues. Finally, Anne Chamberlain describes several aspects of the rehabilitation process which, by using a team approach, embraces the whole breadth of rheumatology.

The 'Interfaces in Medicine' conference on rheumatology was stimulating, informative and enjoyable. We hope this volume communicates some of these feelings to those general practitioners and general physicians who could not be there on the day.

Ian Lewin
Carol Seymour

Contents

1 | Osteoarthritis

Paul Dieppe
Rheumatology Unit, Bristol Royal Infirmary

Osteoarthritis (OA) is an important cause of chronic pain and physical disability. There is no magical cure for it, no expensive investigation and no exciting complication requiring hospital expertise. It affects enormous numbers of people, particularly in the older age groups. The vast majority of sufferers look to their GP for help and advice, and for relief of their symptoms and handicap.

In the past, the lack of exciting interventions or life threatening problems has led to a somewhat negative attitude towards OA. It has been recognised that if a joint falls to pieces, as occurs in a minority of cases, it can be replaced by an orthopaedic surgeon. This has been seen not only as a last resort but also as the only thing that can be done. The attitude has been prevalent that the patient has to 'earn' a joint replacement by years of suffering during which time the doctor has little to offer. Contrary to this belief, there are many simple, effective things which can be done for patients with OA, apart from surgery, and our better understanding of this condition is now doing much to dispel old views.

Discovering the exact cause of pain and disability in an individual presents an interesting diagnostic challenge and, as in all forms of medicine, attention to detail in management can be very rewarding. The knee and hip are the two sites which cause most of the burden of suffering arising from OA, so greatest reference will be made to these two joints.

Defining osteoarthritis: pathology or pain?

OA is often defined as a condition of synovial joints, characterised by focal areas of loss of articular cartilage combined with increased growth and activity of the marginal and subchondral bone. This definition has the advantage that it bears some relationship to the radiographic appearance: severe cartilage loss and bony changes will show on x-ray as joint space narrowing and osteophytosis.

However, there are serious disadvantages to a pathological approach to the definition. As well as hiding the enigmatic and heterogeneous nature of OA, this definition cannot be easily applied in practice. It bears little relationship to the pain and disability which affects the patients. The concept of OA has now changed to the point where it is no longer considered a single disease entity, but rather a pathophysiological state of 'joint failure', representing the final common pathway of many causes and disease processes. As a result, a more pragmatic view of the definition is emerging, varying approaches being used by different interested parties.

Epidemiologists need a simple tool for case definition and tend to rely upon radiographic evidence of altered joint anatomy. X-rays of populations have shown that OA is very common and related to age, and also that different risk factors are linked to different joints. For example, obesity in women is strongly associated with OA of the knee but not the hip.[1] Rheumatologists think of OA as a set of disease processes going on within a joint: a battle between destruction and attempted or aberrant repair.[2] Biomechanical forces can result in more damage to a joint surface and can also activate the repair process. The processes of degradation and repair of cartilage matrix are both biochemically controlled, suggesting that greater understanding of their mechanisms might lead to ways of measuring and also treating OA in individual joints.[3,4] General practitioners see older people with painful joints and theirs is a different perspective, relating most directly to the needs of the community.

Why is osteoarthritis sometimes troublesome?

Patients with evidence of OA on X-ray are often asymptomatic but they are still more likely to have joint pain than those without radiological changes. Even so, there is a discrepancy between epidemiological evidence of joint damage and the experience of pain or disability in the community. This is because the static anatomical changes on the radiograph are not directly related to any part of the OA process which causes pain or altered joint function. Cartilage, which bears the brunt of the pathological changes described, has no nerves. The loss of cartilage thickness and marginal growth of bone seen on an X-ray do not necessarily lead to significant alteration in joint function. This leads to two fascinating questions: what are the causes of pain in OA and what are the causes of disability?

Surprisingly little is known about the real causes of joint pain but it seems that several different processes can be involved.[5] In some cases there is an increase in subchondral bone pressure which can lead to pain at rest and at night. The immediate pain relief after operations such as osteotomy is probably due to reduction of this intra-osseous pressure. In other cases, growth of osteophytes can cause pain and tenderness at joint margins. Other causes of pain include stretching of capsule and ligaments as the anatomy of the joint is disturbed, as well as secondary synovitis or bursitis around the joint. Recent research has emphasised the importance of psychosocial factors in the pain experienced by patients with OA.[6] Many of these causes of pain are transitory and treatable.

Even less is known about the causes of disability in OA although some are obvious and some are also treatable. The degree of disability varies enormously and depends on the sites and severity of disease as well as psychosocial and other circumstances. Severe disturbance of joint anatomy leads to a reduced range of joint motion and to difficulty initiating movement. The stiffness and functional difficulties which many people experience are caused by this. Muscle weakness around the affected joints is also very important and, in one analysis, emerged as the main determinant of disability in patients with OA of the knee.[7] Deformity, particularly if there is secondary ligamentous instability, is another important cause of disability. Pain is a major contributory factor which may be worsened by the increasing social isolation, depression and demoralisation which can go with the discomfort and slowing up experienced by many older people with OA. It is also important to remember that OA may be only one of a number of different factors leading to handicap. Joint disease may become tolerable, for example, if failing eyesight is improved.

What is the differential diagnosis?

Diagnostic difficulty may arise when an older patient first presents with joint pain. There is likely to be evidence of OA, both clinically and radiographically, but is this the cause of pain? In OA, the symptomatic joint is usually marked by inactivity stiffness and use-related pain, worst at the end of the day. Although several joints may be affected, it is usually only one or two sites which dominate the clinical picture. On examination there is a firm swelling at the margins of the joint, a reduced range of motion with pain at the end of the range, crepitus and perhaps evidence of mild inflammation. Muscle wasting around the joint is usually apparent and there may be a number of tender spots around or in the proximity of the joint margin. Other causes of localised joint pain include soft tissue and periarticular problems unrelated to OA, as well as referred pain, from the back for example, and other forms of joint disease such as gout or pseudogout. Generalised joint pain is unlikely to be due to OA, and fibromyalgia, polymyalgia rheumatica, thyroid disease and psychological factors are amongst the many conditions which may need to be considered.

Natural history

Little is known about the preclinical phase of OA but there may be years of asymptomatic development before it becomes a clinical problem. The onset of symptoms is usually gradual and the pain and stiffness of a joint may 'creep up' over months or years. In some cases the onset of pain is acute, sometimes with overt swelling or inflammation of the joint. The subsequent clinical course suggests a phasic disease process, episodes of change being interspersed with long periods, sometimes a decade or more, of stability in which symptoms improve and there is little or no change in the joint anatomy. In many patients it seems as if the reparative process achieves a position of relative control and the joint, although altered in function, is then stable. Patients are then able to adapt to the discomfort, reduced movement and stiffness, resulting in a relative improvement in quality of life. Occasionally there is spontaneous recovery of the altered joint anatomy as well as improvement in the clinical picture. Certainly, not all joints affected by OA are likely to undergo inexorable, slow progression. However, progression will occur in some cases. In the minority who come to surgery there is usually a relatively short period of worsening, severe symptoms occurring for only a year or so prior to operation. This suggests that the joint has gone into a fairly sudden phase of dominant joint destruction, sometimes after a phase of stability.

Much more needs to be known about the natural history of OA and the factors controlling it. There are very few published prospective studies but what data there are suggest that many cases will be better 5–10 years after first being diagnosed.[2] It is therefore inappropriate to advise patients that they will inevitably get worse.

Management of osteoarthritis

Successful management depends upon a good knowledge and understanding of OA and its likely natural history. All forms of treatment benefit from attention to detail such as the dominant causes of pain, the degree of disability and other problems specific to the patient as an individual. A careful history and examination should reveal the main issues, whether they be psychosocial, peri-articular, bony, or otherwise. It should then be possible to provide a combination of useful treatments for a given individual.

Education and patient contact

Many patients with OA just need to know the diagnosis and to be told that they are not wearing out their joints and that it is good to keep active. Occasional patient contact, education and encouragement of this sort can have a markedly beneficial effect on the burden of pain and disability.[5,8]

Physical activity and physiotherapy

Muscle weakness can be a major cause of disability in OA. Early and regular muscle exercises, to strengthen muscles and hence to keep joints stable and protected, are very important in pain relief and the prevention of long-term problems. Physiotherapists can also help patients to maintain a full range of movement and thus preserve optimum function in affected joints. Simple graded exercises are also of benefit in OA. Patients enrolled into an exercise programme fare much better than those left without this encouragement to increase their daily activity. Patients with OA should keep as active as possible.[9]

Sticks, supports and shoes

The provision of a walking stick illustrates that some of the best management strategies for OA are apparently very simple. However, to get good results the stick needs to have the right length and ferrule, it needs to be held in the correct hand and patients need to be shown how to use it properly. A walking stick may improve walking distance and decrease pain considerably. Whilst knee instability may need support, many patients with knee pain also find that supports or bandages give relief as well as a feeling of security. Taping the patella medially, to take pressure off an osteoarthritic patello-femoral facet, also reduces pain and improves function, emphasising again the potential value of simple mechanical interventions in knee OA.[10] Attention to footwear is important and patients should be encouraged to use shoe insoles made from sorbithane or other materials which reduce the high velocity impact loading of joints which occurs at heel strike. Many patients find 'trainers' very comfortable. Any inequality in leg length should also be corrected by heel raises and specially adapted footwear may help with hallux valgus or rigidus. Other orthoses can also be of value according to individual circumstances.

Weight loss

Obesity is an important risk factor for the development of knee OA and weight loss reduces this risk.[11] Weight loss also seems important for obese people with established OA, reducing pain, decreasing the risk of progressive joint damage, increasing mobility and improving general fitness and health.

Rubefacients and other local applications

Many people with OA apply heat or rubefacients to affected joints. Recently, their options for this type of treatment have increased with the introduction of creams and gels containing nonsteroidal anti-inflammatory drugs (NSAIDs). Other topical agents, such as capsaicin, are also being tested.[12] There are many advantages to this kind of self-medication as local applications of any sort will usually give a good deal of pain relief, nearly all of them are safe and they also provide patients with a measure of control over their disease.

Systemic drug therapy

In the first instance patients with painful lower limb OA, who have no obvious periarticular, psychogenic or referred cause for pain, need advice about weight loss, exercise, footwear and perhaps walking aids. Education, patient contact and reassurance can be surprisingly effective.[8] The next step might be simple analgesics taken as required or regularly, such as paracetamol alone or in combinations with dextropropoxyphene. If significant symptoms persist attention should be focused again on local therapy and simple biomechanical interventions, as well as on the use of other drugs. A large number of oral NSAIDs are prescribed in this situation but their use remains controversial. Although of proven benefit for symptoms it is not clear whether they are much better than simple analgesics for most patients.[13-15] The increased risks of gastrointestinal, renal and other side effects are of particular concern in elderly women who are most likely to be suffering from OA. In patients with normal renal function, no history of peptic ulceration and therefore a low risk of side effects, a short trial of NSAIDs is reasonable. If this fails, or if NSAIDs are contraindicated, other options should be considered, such as low dose amitriptyline at night or even acupuncture and other complimentary techniques if these are available locally.

Surgery

A small number of patients with OA do develop severe pain with progressive joint damage. They will generally benefit from surgery, usually a total joint replacement. The indications for surgery have not been established but pain, particularly at night, plus advanced radiographic changes, appear to be the criteria on which most surgeons decide to operate. Severe disability, a major effect on life, such as threatened work, and compromised sexual function should also be considered as reasons for operating. In short, if the patient cannot walk, work or sleep, surgery should be considered.

Conclusion

OA cannot be cured but much can be achieved through careful attention to detail, by analysing the causes of pain and assessing other problems faced by the individual patient. A wide variety of safe interventions can be combined to support, educate and improve patients, thus increasing their quality of life.

References

1. Felson DT. Epidemiology of hip and knee osteoarthritis. *Epidemiol Rev* 1988; **10**: 1–28.
2. Bland JH, Cooper SM. Osteoarthritis: a review of the cell biology involved and evidence for reversibility. *Semin Arthritis Rheum* 1984; **14**: 106–33.
3. Dieppe PA. Osteoarthritis: clinical and research perspective. *Br J Rheumatol* 1991; **30 Suppl 1**: 1–4.
4. Dieppe PA. Some recent clinical approaches to osteoarthritis research. *Semin Arthritis Rheum* 1990; 20 (**3 Suppl 1**): 2–11.
5. McCarthy C, Cushnaghan J, Dieppe PA. Osteoarthritis. In: Wall P, Melzack R, eds. *Pain. 3rd edn.* London: Churchill Livingstone, 1993: in press.
6. Summers MN, Haley WE, Reveille JO, Alarcon GS. Radiographic assessment and psychological variables as predictors of pain and functional impairment in osteoarthritis of the knee and hip. *Arthritis Rheum* 1988; **31**: 204–9.
7. McAlindon T, Cooper C, Kirwan JR. Determinants of disability in osteoarthritis of the knee. *Ann Rheum Dis* 1993; **52**: 258–62.

8. Weinberger M, Tierney WM, Booher P, Katz BP. The impact of increased contact on psychosocial outcomes of patients with osteoarthritis; a randomised controlled trial. *J Rheumatol* 1991; **18**: 849–54.

9. Kovar PA, Allegrante JP, MacKenzie R, Peterson MG, Gutin B, Charlson ME. Supervised fitness walking in patients with osteoarthritis of the knee. *Ann Intern Med* 1992; **116**: 529–34.

10. Cushnaghan J, McCarthy C, Dieppe P. Taping the patella medially: a new treatment for osteoarthritis? *Br J Rheumatol* 1991; **18**: 849–54.

11. Felson DT, Zhang Y, Anthony JM, Naimark A, Anderson JJ. Weight loss reduced the risk for symptomatic knee osteoarthritis in women. The Framingham study. *Ann Intern Med* 1992; **116**: 535–9.

12. McCarthy G, McCarty DJ. Effect of topical capsaicin in the therapy of painful osteoarthritis of the hand. *J Rheumatol* 1992; **19**: 604–7.

13. Bradley JD, Brandt KD, Katz BP, Kalazinki MPH, Ryan SI. Comparison of an anti-inflammatory dose of ibuprofen, an analgesic dose of ibuprofen and acetaminophen in the treatment of patients with osteoarthritis of the knee. *N Engl J Med* 1991; **325**: 87–91.

14. McAlindon TE, Dieppe PA. The medical management of osteoarthritis of the knee: an inflammatory issue? *Br J Rheumatol* 1990; **29**: 471–3.

15. Dieppe PA, Frankel SJ, Toth B. Is research into the treatment of osteoarthritis with non-steroidal anti-inflammatory drugs misdirected? *Lancet* 1993; **341**: 353–4.

2 | Hyperuricaemia and gout

J Thomas Scott

Charing Cross Hospital and Kennedy Institute of Rheumatology, London

Chronic hyperuricaemia is far more common in men than women and in many cases it remains asymptomatic throughout life. In perhaps 10% of cases, notably in middle-aged and elderly men, it results in symptomatic gout, provoked by the inflammatory response to monosodium urate crystals in and around joints. Typically it presents as recurrent self-limiting attacks of acute arthritis in one or two joints, usually in the lower limb and especially in the big toe, where it causes severe pain, tenderness, swelling and redness. This is followed by gradual resolution into asymptomatic intervals, intercritical gout, usually lasting from 6 months to two years. Before modern treatments this might have led to greater or lesser degrees of permanent joint damage and to deposits of urate in the pinna of the ear and elsewhere.[1] The clinical picture is variable and now includes an increasing number of elderly women on diuretic treatment, particularly with impaired renal function, some of whom present with subacute polyarticular disease which may be misdiagnosed as osteo- or rheumatoid arthritis.[2] Occasionally, such patients give no history of acute attacks but develop tophi in association with Heberden's nodes at the distal interphalangeal joints.[3]

Pathophysiology

The purines, adenine and guanine, are metabolised to hypoxanthine and xanthine respectively and are then catalysed by xanthine oxidase to uric acid. In plasma, uric acid is almost completely ionised as sodium urate, reaching saturation at 420 μmol/l. The normal range is about 180–420 μmol/l for men and 120–360 μmol/l for women, hence the risk of urate precipitation. Urate is freely filtered by the glomeruli and is almost totally reabsorbed by the proximal tubules. Uric acid is then secreted, also by the proximal tubule, so that two thirds of the daily urate production is finally cleared via the kidneys.

At any given time, the plasma level of urate is a function of production and clearance rates. Because of this, hyperuricaemia has sometimes been described as 'primary' or 'metabolic' if there is a high production rate, and 'renal' if there is reduced clearance. This classification into 'over producers' and 'under excreters' is a useful concept as long as one appreciates that both mechanisms may operate in the same patient, and in some conditions the mechanisms may not be known. Decreased urate clearance contributes to hyperuricaemia in the great majority of patients with gout.[4]

Management of acute gout

Acute gout is usually suspected because of its typical clinical picture. If this is present, a high serum urate, above 420 μmol/l in men and 360 μmol/l in women, makes the diagnosis highly likely. Gout with a persistently normal serum uric acid is rare unless urate-lowering drug have recently been used. If there is doubt, and if infection is also a possibility, the joint should be aspirated. In 85% of cases the fluid contains intracellular or extracellular needle-shaped crystals of sodium urate, 2 to 10 μm in length, which on polarised light microscopy with a first-order red compensator show negative birefringence.

Acute gout is self-limiting, lasting from a few hours to several weeks, but usually for more than seven days if left untreated. Immediate treatment is directed towards rapid relief of inflammation so effective anti-inflammatory drugs should be started as soon as possible. Nonsteroidal anti-inflammatory drugs (NSAIDs) are now the treatment of choice, colchicine has a smaller place and corticosteroids are used only in exceptional circumstances. Aspirin is not used because low doses increase serum urate and higher doses of over 3 gm daily, although they increase urate excretion, do not ease symptoms. Urate lowering drugs play no part in the management of acute gout but they are relevant to long-term management. They should not be started during an attack but patients already taking them should continue, otherwise, an attack may be aggravated and prolonged.[5]

Nonsteroidal anti-inflammatory drugs

NSAIDs are the treatment of choice for acute gout: indomethacin 50 mg 3–4 times daily by mouth, or 100 mg twice daily by suppository, for 5–8 days is effective in the majority of patients. Other NSAIDs may also be used, for example: naproxen 500 mg twice daily; ibuprofen 600 mg four times daily; ketoprofen 50 mg four times daily; sulindac 200 mg twice daily; tolmetin sodium 600 mg four times daily; diclofenac sodium 50 mg three times daily or piroxicam 20 mg once daily. Response may be strikingly prompt if the drug is given in maximum initial doses as early as possible during the acute attack. More than 90% of patients experience great pain relief within one day and complete resolution of the attack within 5–8 days. Patients known to be at risk often benefit from a supply of tablets at home, to take according to written instructions at the first suggestion of an attack. With this approach it is often possible to terminate an acute episode within three days.

Colchicine

Colchicine, one of the oldest remedies for gout, is most effective if used within 24 hours of onset of an attack. Because of its tendency to cause nausea, abdominal pain and diarrhoea it is used mainly when NSAIDs are poorly tolerated or contraindicated, for example in patients on warfarin or in cardiac or renal failure. It should not be used if there is biliary obstruction or if creatinine clearance is less than 10 ml per minute. It is given orally at a dose of 1.0 mg initially followed by 0.5 mg up to a maximum of every 2–3 hours until joint pain has resolved, until the total dose has reached 10 mg or until side effects occur. In the elderly, 0.5 mg twice daily is often satisfactory. The course should not be repeated within three days.

Corticosteroids

Corticosteroids are rarely used for acute gout but they have a place in severe polyarticular attacks where NSAIDs and colchicine are ineffective or contraindicated. Prednisolone can be used in doses of 20–40 mg daily for 1–3 days followed by gradual reduction to avoid a rebound attack. Intra-articular steroid injections may also be used in patients who are unable to take tablets, for example postoperatively or because of gastrointestinal disease.

Investigation of hyperuricaemia

In the obese middle-aged man presenting with a typical clinical history, a high plasma urate makes a diagnosis of gout extremely likely and it is arguable to what extent further investigation is needed. A drug history is important and simple laboratory investigation will exclude blood dyscrasias and renal impairment. A

confident diagnosis is helpful if long-term therapy is to be given
and this can be made if urate crystals are present in a joint aspirate.
Attention should then be quickly transferred to issues such as obesity, hypertension, hyperlipidaemia and the cardiovascular disease to
which such patients are prone.[4]

The possibility of provoking factors should always be considered.
Various diuretics decrease urate excretion, such as : thiazides, chlor-
thalidone, frusemide, acetazolamide, triamterene and amiloride.
Other drugs which decrease uric acid excretion include: aspirin,
pyrazinamide, nicotinic acid, ethambutol and l-dopa. Urate production is increased by fructose, nicotinic acid, vitamin B12 injections, cytotoxic drugs and pancreatic extract. Regular ethanol
consumption increases urate synthesis and the acidosis of acute
intoxication inhibits excretion.[6] Hyperuricaemia has also been associated with lead poisoning (saturnine gout), starvation, diabetic
ketoacidosis, lactic acidosis, Down's syndrome, acromegaly, hypothyroidism, hyperparathyroidism, psoriasis, sarcoid and Bartter's
syndrome.[7]

Gout should be assessed with care if it presents in men before the
age of 30 and in women before the menopause. A family history is
likely, the more so the younger the age of presentation. Attacks of
gout tend to be frequent and urolithiasis becomes a problem unless
effective treatment is given early. Serum urate is always raised but
the diagnosis should be confirmed by aspiration of an affected
joint. Additional investigations should include measurement of uric
acid production and excretion rates. The 24 hour urinary uric acid
excretion can be used as an index of uric acid production rate and
this can be measured on two consecutive days after 5 days on a low
purine alcohol and caffeine free diet. Foods to be avoided during
this time include sweetbreads, pâté, liver, kidney, fish roe, herrings,
shellfish, tinned fish, sardines, anchovies, mussels and meat extracts
such as soups and gravies. There should also be a reduction in
meats, other fish, beans, lentils and peas. Overproduction is indicated by a 24h uric acid excretion rate in excess of 3.8 mmol on a
restricted diet or, if this is impractical, 5.5 mmol on a standard diet.
The renal handling of uric acid can be assessed by various simple
techniques. A urinary uric acid to creatinine ratio of over 0.8
suggests overproduction but this screening test can be misleading.
The ratio of urate clearance to creatinine clearance is more satisfactory and values of 7% or less indicate undersecretion. Up to three
quarters of patients with early onset gout, including most of the
women, will have reduced urate clearance, a fifth will have evidence
of increased uric acid production and the occasional case will have

chronic haemolytic anaemia, lead exposure or a syndrome with a defect in renal handling.[8]

In a small minority of cases there will be a specific enzyme defect leading to marked purine overproduction. Complete deficiency of hypoxanthine guanine phosphoribosyltransferase (HGPRT) causes the X-linked recessive Lesch-Nyhan syndrome. In addition to hyperuricaemia and gout, affected males also have mental retardation, basal ganglia dysfunction, spasticity and a tendency to self-mutilation. Partial deficiency of HGPRT and overactivity of phosphoribosylpyrophosphate (PRPP) synthetase also result in gout and renal calculi in the second or third decade. Glucose-6-phosphatase and partial aldolase-beta deficiency may also be implicated. Purine enzyme activity needs to be assessed using specialised techniques. If a genetic cause for hyperuricaemia and gout is identified, family members should be screened so that affected but asymptomatic cases can be offered early treatment to prevent acute gout and renal impairment.

Management of chronic hyperuricaemia

Asymptomatic hyperuricaemia

The risks of mild asymptomatic hyperuricaemia, without a history of overt gout, have previously been exaggerated. The chance of getting gout is relatively small and it can be treated if it occurs, after which long term prophylaxis can then be considered. A link has been suggested between hyperuricaemia and cardiovascular disease but there now seems no direct relationship. In the past there has been anxiety about the adverse effects of asymptomatic hyperuricaemia on the kidney but, in practice, the risk of renal failure is the same as for the general population. The risk of renal calculi is also small enough to adopt a policy of waiting for the first stone before starting drug treatment.[5]

Mild degrees of asymptomatic hyperuricaemia are best managed by life-style modification. Obesity is common in hyperuricaemic patients and weight reduction lowers serum urate. Dietary restriction should be realistic and consistent and should generally involve a reduction in foods high in purines. Health foods containing high quantities of yeast, ascorbic acid and nicotinic acid should be avoided and alcohol should be reduced to a minimum. A moderate amount of exercise is almost certainly beneficial.[4]

Opinions differ about the management of asymptomatic hyperuricaemia if the plasma urate is elevated above 540 µmol/l. This finding is usually associated with an underlying cause. In chronic renal failure it is usually treated with allopurinol, small doses producing an adequate fall in uric acid but larger doses often causing a skin rash. Rarely it results from an inherited enzyme defect such as partial HGPRT deficiency when it will need lifelong treatment to avoid complications.

Symptomatic hyperuricaemia

For symptomatic hyperuricaemia, indications for lowering the serum urate vary to some extent with individual cases. Elderly patients with atypical gout present a particular problem in management where predisposing factors, such as diuretics, cannot be avoided. With a moderately raised serum urate and after perhaps one or two mild attacks of gout, many patients prefer to modify their life styles, avoiding long-term tablet treatment but reconsidering the position after further attacks. In general, treatment should be started if attacks of gout are more frequent than two or three times a year, if there are chronic joint changes or tophi or if there is evidence of renal damage. Treatment is also prudent if gout is associated with a consistently high serum urate concentration, perhaps above 540 μmol/l, because the disease is then usually progressive in terms of frequency of attacks and chronic joint damage.

Serum urate can be lowered effectively by reducing its production rate with allopurinol or by increasing excretion with the uricosuric drugs, probenecid and sulphinpyrazone. In principle it would seem that overproducers of uric acid should be treated with allopurinol and underexcreters with uricosuric drugs. In practice the majority of patients with gout show reduced clearance of uric acid but they also do well on allopurinol so it is increasingly the drug of choice.

Allopurinol

Similar to hypoxanthine in structure, allopurinol acts as a competitive inhibitor of xanthine oxidase, preventing the conversion of hypoxanthine to xanthine and finally xanthine to uric acid. It also reduces purine synthesis by several different mechanisms. The result is an increase in the more soluble oxypurines, hypoxanthine and xanthine. Serum urate levels fall within 2 days of starting treatment and often become normal in 7–24 days. Attacks of gout usually stop within 3–6 months on continuous therapy and tophi may dissolve over 6–24 months.

Care is needed in the early phase of treatment because an unduly sharp reduction in urate may provoke, by some unknown mechanism, frequent and severe attacks of gout. Although this may occur in less than a quarter of cases it may be prudent to offer NSAIDs to cover the first 3–6 months of therapy whilst continuing with allopurinol as planned. It should be started at a dose as low as 100 mg daily, increasing gradually according to serum urate levels. In the elderly, especially if there is any degree of renal impairment, it could be started at as low a dose as 100 mg on alternate days. The dose needed to maintain serum urate within the normal range varies from 200–800 mg daily and is usually 300–400 mg daily. If it is then discontinued, serum urate rises rapidly to pretreatment levels although recurrence of gout may not occur for long periods.

The half-life of allopurinol is only 1–3 hours but that of oxypurinol, its active metabolite, is 16–20 hours, so it can be given once daily. Oxypurinol is cleared by the kidneys so the dose of allopurinol should be reduced in renal failure, to as little as 50 mg on alternate days. Thiazide diuretics interfere with the excretion of oxypurinol, leading to further elevation in plasma levels. Side-effects of allopurinol occur in just over 3% of cases, the commonest being a skin rash, particularly in renal failure when it correlates with high blood levels of oxypurinol. Desensitisation may be attempted by reintroducing the drug at very low doses, but this is not always successful. Adverse interactions may occur with other drugs. For example, the effect of warfarin is potentiated, ampicillin rashes may be increased threefold and there is a greater chance of bone marrow suppression with cyclophosphamide. Azathioprine and 6-mercaptopurine need to be reduced to a quarter of their usual doses because their inactivation pathway via xanthine oxidase is blocked.

Allopurinol is most valuable in gout associated with extensive tophi, acute and chronic urate nephropathy and severe renal failure. It is particularly indicated for the rare genetic disorders with marked overproduction of uric acid and for secondary hyperuricaemiain following treatment of leukaemia or lymphoma.[5]

Uricosuric drugs

Uricosuric drugs increase the clearance of urate by inhibiting renal tubular reabsorption. They are effective drugs although now used in a minority of cases because of the efficacy of allopurinol. Potentially, 75% of patients are able to respond to such therapy with normalisation of serum urate, resolution of gout attacks and dissolution of tophi. Failure in the remaining 25% results from antagonism by salicylates, lack of efficacy if creatinine clearance is below 30–50 ml/min and uncommonly from adverse effects such as anorexia, nausea, vomiting or skin rashes. As with allopurinol, but to a lesser degree, acute gout may be provoked by the early phase of uricosuric treatment so NSAIDs may be helpful for the first few months. To minimise the risk of acute gout, and to prevent formation of renal calculi associated with the initial rise in urate excretion, uricosuric drugs should be started at low dose and increased over several weeks. In addition, urinary volume should be at least two litres daily and in those at special risk of stone formation the urine should be alkalinised with sodium bicarbonate 2–6 gm daily or acetazolamide 500 mg daily.

Probenecid is given initially at a dose of 250 mg twice daily, increasing to a maximum of 3 gm daily according to response. Sulphinpyrazone is given initially at a dose of 50–100 mg twice daily and gradually increased, if needed, to a maximum of 800 mg daily. Benzbromarone is another potent uricosuric drug which can be obtained for individual patients. It is effective in the presence of impaired renal function[9] and can be tried in patients who develop a skin rash with allopurinol.

Specific indications for uricosuric drugs include allergy or intolerance to allopurinol and the rare cases with massive tophaceous gout where combined treatment with allopurinol may be necessary. Special care is needed in this situation because of the probability of coincident renal impairment. In addition, probenecid used with allopurinol may block the tubular reabsorption of oxypurinol, thus increasing its excretion and reducing its effectiveness as a urate lowering agent.

Conclusion

Gout is one of the most easily treated of the rheumatic diseases. It is usually diagnosed by the typical history, clinical findings and raised serum urate, but certainty is greater if urate crystals are demonstrated in joint aspirate. The increasing incidence of atypical gout, particularly in elderly women, should be borne in mind to avoid delay in diagnosis and effective treatment.

Acute attacks of gout respond well to NSAIDs and, where these are contraindicated, colchicine is a useful alternative. Urate lowering drugs should not be started during acute attacks but they should be continued by patients already taking them. Conditions which are common in gouty patients, such as obesity, hypertension, hyperlipidaemia and ischaemic heart disease, should be evaluated and actively treated.

Mild hyperuricaemia which is asymptomatic or which only causes occasional episodes of gout may be treated by life style modification. More marked hyperuricaemia, with repeated attacks of gout, gouty nephropathy or risk of these, should be treated with urate lowering drugs. These should be started at low dose or in combination with NSAIDs to avoid the chance of acute gout early in the treatment. In renal failure uricosuric agents are ineffective and allopurinol should be used with caution.

Detailed biochemical investigation, sometimes at specialist centres, may be necessary for certain patient groups, notably young men and premenopausal women with marked hyperuricaemia, gout or a positive family history.

References

1. Scott JT. Gout. In: Scott JT, ed. *Copeman's textbook of the rheumatic diseases. 6th edn.* Edinburgh: Churchill Livingstone, 1986: 883–937.
2. Borg EJJ, Rasher JJ. Gout in the elderly: a separate entity? *Ann Rheum Dis* 1987; **46**: 72–6.
3. Hollingsworth P, Scott JT, Burry HC. Non-articular gout: hyperuricaemia and tophus formation without gouty arthritis. *Arthritis Rheum* 1983; **26**: 98–101.
4. Scott JT. Gout. *Baillière's Clin Rheumatol* 1987; **1**: 525–46.
5. Fam AG. Strategies and controversies in the treatment of gout and hyperuricaemia. *Baillière's Clin Rheumatol* 1990; **4**: 177–92.
6. Scott JT. Drug-induced gout. *Baillière's Clin Rheumatol* 1991; **5**: 39–60.
7. German DC, Holmes EW. Hyperuricaemia and gout. *Med Clin North Am* 1986; **70**: 419–36.
8. Dieppe PA. Investigation and management of gout in the young and the elderly. *Ann Rheum Dis* 1991; **50**: 263–6.
9. Delbarre F, Auscher C, Saporta L, DGery A, Danchot J. Treatment of gout with a dibrom derivative of benzopuranes. *Rev Rhum Mal Osteoartic* 1973; **40**: 275–7.

3 | Polymyalgia rheumatica and giant cell arteritis

Brian L Hazleman
Addenbrooke's Hospital, Cambridge and Newmarket Hospital

Polymyalgia rheumatica (PMR) and giant cell arteritis (GCA) occur almost entirely in white populations but the same diseases have been recognised occasionally in black Americans and also world-wide. They are seldom diagnosed below the age of 50 years, peak incidence occurs between ages 60–75 and three times as many women are affected as men. There is a genetic association with HLA–DR4.

Clinical features

In the elderly patient with muscle pain, stiffness, constitutional symptoms and a raised erythrocyte sedimentation rate (ESR), the diagnosis of PMR is partly one of exclusion and the differential diagnosis is wide because of other conditions which it can simulate. In many cases, patients and their doctors initially attribute symptoms to degenerative joint disease or even to psychological illness. In others, the systemic features and laboratory abnormalities may lead to extensive investigation for infective endocarditis, carcinoma, myeloma, leukaemia and lymphoma. PMR can usually be differentiated from late onset rheumatoid arthritis by the absence of prominent peripheral joint pain and swelling, although in some patients it may show clinical and histological features of a mild proximal synovitis. There is little evidence to suggest that the musculoskeletal symptoms of PMR are related to vasculitis. It can also be distinguished from polymositis because movement is limited predominantly by pain rather than by muscular weakness. In practice, non-specific clinical features, the frequent absence of physical signs and the process of investigation may result in a delay of several months before a firm diagnosis of PMR is made.[1]

GCA should be considered in any patient over the age of 50 years with recent onset of headache, transient or sudden loss of vision, myalgia, unexplained fever or anaemia or high ESR. Symptoms, in

the majority of cases, result from arteritis of the scalp or eye whilst
jaw pain on eating is caused by arteritis of the temporal, maxillary
and facial arteries.[2] Visual loss usually results from optic nerve
ischaemia and more rarely from retinal artery occlusion and other
lesions.[3] In a minority of cases large vessels may also be affected
causing myocardial infarction, stroke, intermittent claudication of
arms or legs and aortic dissection. Because symptoms and signs may
be transient and vary in severity, patients should be questioned
carefully about recent as well as current symptoms. The arteries of
the head, neck and limbs should be examined for tenderness,
enlargement, thrombosis and bruits. It is not usually difficult to
separate GCA from other forms of arteritis. It rarely, if ever, affects
the kidneys, it is serologically distinct from systemic lupus erythematosus and none of the other vasculitides, with the exception
of Wegener's granulomatosis and occasionally polyarteritis nodosa
(PAN) has such a marked effect on the cranial arteries.

There is a complex relationship between PMR and GCA. Paulley
& Hughes in 1960[4] were the first to link them, suggesting that PMR
was a prodromal manifestation of temporal arteritis. Certainly they
share many similarities such as age and sex distribution, biopsy
findings and laboratory features, even though these may simply
reflect non-specific inflammatory changes. Both conditions are
now considered to form a disease spectrum and they may occur
together in the same individual. PMR is sometimes viewed as a condition which runs a prolonged or recurring course, in contrast to
GCA which tends to manifest mostly as a single episode of vasculitis.
In some cases, symptoms of PMR may precede or follow those of
GCA, usually within 1-6 years but sometimes with an interval of up
to 10 years. In addition, of those patients with PMR who have no
symptoms or signs of GCA, 10-15% will have positive temporal
artery biopsies[5] and the clinical characteristics of these cases are no
different from those with a negative biopsy. Even so, many patients
with PMR show no evidence of arteritis even if followed up for many
years. Conversely, patients with GCA, even when large vessels are
involved, often do not develop PMR.

Investigations

In more than 95% of untreated cases of both PMR and GCA the
ESR is usually greatly elevated, far more than might occur in otherwise healthy elderly people, and this provides a useful means of
monitoring therapy. However, a normal ESR is occasionally found
in patients with active biopsy-proven disease.[6] A mild hypochromic

or a more marked normochromic anaemia is common, it may be the presenting feature and it resolves with treatment.[7] Leucocyte and differential counts are generally normal, as is the platelet count, although this may sometimes be increased. Alkaline phosphatase and hepatic transaminases may be raised whilst protein electrophoresis may show a non-specific rise in alpha-2 globulin with less frequent elevation of alpha-1 and gamma globulins. Measurement of acute phase proteins, alpha-1 antitrypsin, orosomucoid, haptoglobin and C-reactive protein tend to parallel ESR and are no more helpful than ESR in the assessment of disease activity.[8]

In PMR temporal artery biopsies are not necessary if clinical evidence for GCA is absent, if symptoms are mild and of recent onset, or if they are stable and of long duration. Such patients can be followed closely without biopsy as there is little risk of blindness. Muscle biopsy is rarely necessary but may show type 2 fibre atrophy. Evidence of vasculitis within muscle argues against a diagnosis of PMR and is more in favour of polyarteritis nodosa. Synovial tissue, if it is examined, may show mild inflammatory changes. In GCA a temporal artery biopsy is highly desirable although false-negatives may occur in a third or more of cases, mainly because of the focal nature of the inflammation in the superficial arteries. If temporal artery biopsy is performed, a long segment of a symptomatic or clinically abnormal segment of artery should be chosen.[9] Temporal artery angiography is not helpful as there is no characteristic abnormality and false positives are common, usually because of atheroma.

Management

Corticosteroids improve quality of life for patients with PMR and GCA but there is no evidence that they influence the natural history of the disease. In principle they should be given in sufficient dose to suppress the disease and then reduced to the lowest maintenance dose which controls symptoms and lowers the ESR. Exact recommendations do vary because of the relative lack of clinical trials. The response to steroids is usually dramatic and occurs within days. For PMR prednisolone is often used initially in doses of 10–20 mg daily but some patients show insufficient response on the lower dose. Reducing the daily dose to 5–7.5 mg as early as the second month is also associated with a tendency to relapse.[10]

Corticosteroids are mandatory in the treatment of GCA because they reduce the incidence of blindness and rapidly relieve symptoms, in contrast to nonsteroidal anti-inflammatory drugs

(NSAIDs) which lessen pain but do not prevent arteritic complications. Ideally they should be given after the diagnosis has been confirmed histologically but where GCA is strongly suspected delay should be avoided to prevent the risk of blindness. A temporal artery biopsy performed several days after corticosteroids have been started will still show inflammatory changes. If biopsy of a temporal or other artery is negative but the clinical suspicion of the disease is strong, steroid treatment should be started or continued anyway.

For GCA prednisolone should be used in initial doses of at least 40 mg daily for the first month. Some patients will relapse if the dose is reduced to 20 mg daily after the first five days or if 20 mg daily is used as the initial dose.[10] Some ophthalmologists prefer an initial daily dose of 60 mg or more but this has to be balanced against the potential risks of high dose steroids in the elderly. Fear of vasculitic complications in biopsy-positive GCA sometimes leads to initial doses of up to 100mg daily and occasionally to intravenous steroids. This approach might well be used in patients presenting with visual disturbance and although it is able to arrest further deterioration over a period of several days it does not usually restore lost vision.[3] Once initial symptoms are controlled, reducing the dose of prednisolone is largely a matter of clinical judgment as individual cases vary greatly. A weekly decrements of up to 5 mg would seem reasonable, down to a dose of 10 mg daily. Thereafter a slower reduction of 1 mg every 2-4 weeks might be sufficient. Rapid reduction or withdrawal of steroids is a disadvantage and may even prove fatal.[11]

Significant side effects of steroid treatment may occur in one fifth to one half of patients and these are related to high initial doses, size of maintenance doses, cumulative doses and increased duration of treatment. However, if the initial dose of prednisolone for PMR is 10 mg or less, and if the maintenance dose is 7.5 mg or less, most patients are virtually free from side effects.[12] In some cases, the risk of relapse, particularly with arteritic complications, has to be balanced against the risk of steroid associated side effects. Patients who are unable to reduce the dose of prednisolone because of recurring symptoms or who develop serious steroid related side effects pose particular problems. Azathioprine has been shown to exert a modest steroid sparing effect but methotrexate has not been evaluated adequately.

In the majority of cases, once treatment has been started, disease activity seems to decline steadily but relapse may occur and is more likely during the initial 18 months of treatment and within one year of withdrawal of steroids. Clinical relapse may occur without a rise in ESR and the ESR may rise without corresponding symptoms. There is no reliable method of predicting those most at risk, but arteritic relapse is unusual in patients initially presenting with pure PMR. Temporal artery biopsy does not seem to predict outcome and measurement of acute phase proteins is no more helpful than ESR. In the future, immunological tests may be of some value in predicting when steroids can be withdrawn safely. For example, a study of CD8+ cells, a subset of serum T cells, showed a profound and selective reduction in numbers for up to one year despite symptom control, a normal ESR and normal C-reactive protein on steroid treatment. Numbers had returned to normal after two years.[13]

Controversy exists over the expected duration of treatment for PMR and GCA.[14] For PMR the median duration of treatment at the Mayo Clinic in the USA was 11 months. Three quarters of the patients had stopped taking steroids by two years. For GCA most patients had stopped taking steroids within two years. European experience within the last 20 years suggests that between one third and one half of patients are able to discontinue treatment after 2 years. The consensus seems to be that stopping treatment is easible from two years onwards.

Conclusion

PMR and GCA form a disease spectrum which is satisfying to diagnose and treat.[15] Unpleasant symptoms and serious consequences can be prevented almost entirely by corticosteroid therapy but there is no objective method of determining individual prognosis so decisions concerning duration of treatment remain empirical. Patients should be warned to expect treatment for at least two years whilst most should be able to stop taking steroids after 4–5 years.[16] Monitoring for relapse should continue for 6–12 months after stopping steroids; thereafter patients should be asked to report back urgently if arteritic symptoms occur. The risk of this happening is small and unpredictable but a few patients may need low dose steroid treatment indefinitely.

The overall strategy should be to use an adequate dose of prednisolone for the first month to obtain good symptomatic control with a fall in ESR, then to aim for maintenance doses of less than 10 mg daily after six months. Exact doses will need to be adjusted according to individual need but a possible schedule is prednisolone 15 mg daily for PMR, reducing to about 7.5–10 mg daily by 6–8 weeks. Patient with GCA should be treated with 40 mg daily for the first month unless visual symptoms persist when higher doses of 60–80 mg daily may be needed. A suitable dose reduction would be to 20 mg daily at about 8 weeks. For both PMR and GCA, gradual reduction by 1 mg every 2–3 months can be attempted, with possible withdrawal of steroids after 2 years. Reduction of prednisolone on alternate days once daily doses of less than 5 mg are reached makes withdrawal easier and the addition of NSAIDs may relieve some of the minor muscular symptoms which might occur at this stage. Some patients find it impossible to reduce below a final maintenance dose of prednisolone 2–3 mg daily and this is probably safe to continue.

References

1. Paice EW. Giant cell arteritis: difficult decisions in diagnosis, investigation and treatment. *Postgrad Med J* 1989; **65**: 743–7.
2. Jones JG. Clinical features of giant cell arteritis. *Baillière's Clin Rheumatol* 1991; **5**: 413–30.
3. Hayreh SS. Ophthalmic features of giant cell arteritis. *Baillière's Clin Rheumatol* 1991; **5**: 431–59.
4. Paulley JW, Hughes JP. Giant cell arteritis or arteritis of the aged. *Br Med J* 1960; **2**: 1562–7.
5. Alestig K, Barr J. Giant cell arteritis; biopsy study of polymyalgia rheumatica, including one case of Takayasu's disease. *Lancet* 1963; **1**: 1228–30.
6. Mowat AG, Hazleman BL. Polymyalgia rheumatica: a clinical study with particular reference to arterial disease. *J Rheumatol* 1974; **1**: 190–202.
7. Jones JG, Hazleman BL. Prognosis and management of polymyalgia rheumatica. *Ann Rheum Dis* 1981; **40**: 1–5.
8. Kyle V, Cawston TE, Hazleman BL. ESR and C-reactive protein in the assessment of polymyalgia rheumatica/giant cell arteritis on presentation and during follow up. *Ann Rheum Dis* 1989; **48**: 667–71.
9. Klein GE, Campbell RJ, Hunder GG, Carney JA. Skip lesions in temporal arteritis. *Mayo Clin Proc* 1976; **51**: 504–8.
10. Kyle V, Hazleman BL. Treatment of polymyalgia rheumatica and giant cell arteritis. I. Steroid regimes in the first 2 months. *Ann Rheum Dis* 1989; **48**: 658–61.
11. Nordberg E, Bengtsson BA. Death rates and causes of deaths in 284 consecutive patients with giant cell arteritis confirmed by biopsy. *Br Med J* 1989; **299**: 549–50.
12. Kyle V, Hazleman BL. Treatment of polymyalgia rheumatica and giant cell arteritis. II The relationship between steroid dose and steroid associated side effects. *Ann Rheum Dis* 1989; **48**: 662–6.
13. Dasgupta B, Duke O, Timms AM, Pitzalis C, Panayi GS. Selective depletion and activation of CD8+ lymphocytes from peripheral blood of patients with polymyalgia rheumatica and giant cell arteritis. *Ann*

Rheum Dis 1989; **48**: 307–11.
14. Kyle V, Hazleman BL. Stopping steroids in polymyalgia rheumatica and giant cell arteritis. *Br Med J* 1990; **300**: 344–5.
15. Mason JC, Walport MJ. Giant cell arteritis. *Br Med J* 1992; **305**: 68–9.
16. Anon. The management of polymyalgia rheumatica and giant cell arteritis. *Drug Ther Bull* 1993; **31**: 65-8.

4 | Rheumatic diseases of childhood

Patricia Woo
Clinical Research Centre, Northwick Park Hospital, Harrow

In childhood most minor injuries to muscles, ligaments and joints resolve quickly before a visit to the doctor is considered necessary. The general practitioner is usually consulted if there is more severe injury leading to loss of function or if there is arthritis of recent onset or muscle weakness occurring without obvious cause. Juvenile chronic arthritis (JCA) is rare with an incidence of 0.13–0.19 per 1000,[1,2] and the connective tissue disorders of childhood are even more unusual. For children with these conditions shared care between the primary care physician, and a paediatric rheumatologist provide optimal treatment.

Aches and pains in children

Many of the aches and pains in childhood can be managed by primary care physicians with access to physiotherapy departments but secondary referral to a hospital specialist tends to occur for the following conditions:

- hypermobility syndrome
- growing pains
- chondromalacia patellae and Osgood-Schlatter's disease
- irritable hip
- acute arthritis as a reaction to infection

Hypermobility syndrome

Joint laxity is far more common in children than adults and in the majority of cases it is lost with age. Currently there is no standard method for assessing hypermobility in children but if one applies the Carter and Wilkinson hypermobility score for adults a large number of children fall into this category. The proportion of hypermobile children who develop musculoskeletal symptoms is not known but 39% of our cases with mechanical musculoskeletal problems are hypermobile, suggesting that it is an important factor.

The commonest presenting problem is anterior knee pain and classically the child points to the patella as being painful. The affected knee joint is hyperextendable and sometimes there is also patello-femoral crepitus suggesting a mild degree of chondro-malacia. Such children tend to be very athletic and may also have had a recent growth spurt. Management includes reassurance and physiotherapy with daily exercises to strengthen the muscles controlling joint movement.

Growing pains

During the growth spurt, children often present with peri-articular pains, usually affecting tendinous insertions. Again, the knee is the commonest joint involved and management consists of reassurance and improving muscle strength. Recurrence of enthesitis, especially in children without a history of growth spurt or sports injury, should raise the possibility of juvenile ankylosing spondylitis.

Chondromalacia patellae and Osgood-Schlatter's disease

These conditions also tend to occur in active children who may have just been through a spell of intense athletic activity. Pain and tenderness in the knee are localised to the patella or the tibial tubercle. Physiotherapy usually results in a cure.

Irritable hip

A child with the irritable hip ('transient synovitis of the hip') often presents with a history of upper respiratory tract infection, an extremely painful hip and a limp. Management in general practice is a subject of some discussion but with bed rest most cases settle considerably within 48 hours and subside after one week. If pain persists the child should be referred to an orthopaedic surgeon or a paediatric rheumatologist. If ultrasound reveals an effusion the joint should be aspirated under general anaesthetic to exclude septic arthritis. Traditional management has been bed rest with traction. Like 'growing pains' and ethesitis, recurrence should raise the possibility of chronic arthritic disease, so the child should be referred sooner rather than later to a paediatric rheumatologist or a paediatrician with a special interest in rheumatology.

Acute arthritis as a reaction to infection

Upper respiratory tract and streptococcal throat infections are the usual precipitating events for childhood acute arthritis. The child often has a fever and there may be a variety of rashes as well as one or more swollen joints. The arthritis usually settles within 2 weeks but may grumble on for up to 3 months. It differs from the flitting arthritis of rheumatic fever which presents with very hot, red, swollen, exquisitely tender joints.[3] Nonsteroidal anti-inflammatory drugs (NSAIDs) relieve the discomfort, but salicylates need to be used with caution in children under age 12 yrs because of the possible association with Reye's syndrome. Arthritis persisting in one joint beyond three months, or the involvement of further joints, should alert to the development of juvenile chronic arthritis and the child should by referred to a specialist as soon as possible.

Juvenile chronic arthritis

The nomenclature for juvenile chronic arthritis (JCA), a heterogeneous group of diseases, is under international discussion. The term applies to all chronic arthritides with onset before age 16 yrs and most paediatric rheumatologists use a working classification which depends on the mode of onset within the first 3–6 months.[4,5]

Pauciarticular JCA (4 joints or fewer)

This is the commonest type of JCA which is further subdivided into: *young onset* before age 6 yrs; *older onset* after 6 yrs and both may be described as *extended* if 4 or more joints are involved between 6 and 12 months after onset.

(a) Young onset pauciarticular JCA

Girls are affected much more frequently than boys with a peak onset at 3 yrs. Remission occurs in 80% of cases so management consists of preventing deformities, controlling discomfort and supervising exercises to maintain muscle strength and joint function.

Genetically as well as clinically this is the most homogenous group in that there is a strong association with HLA A2, DR5, DRw6 and DRw8. Approximately 50% of cases have low antinuclear antibody (ANA) titres and within this subgroup 60–80% have silent anterior uveitis. This problem also occurs, but to a lesser extent, in ANA negative children, so three monthly slit lamp examination is essential. In those affected, timely treatment with local steroids can prevent permanent visual loss.

In our series of young onset pauciarticular JCA, more than 4 joints become involved within a year of onset in about 20% of cases. These patients are particularly resistant to second line drugs apart from steroids. However, a recent pilot study suggests that low dose methotrexate may be effective and a placebo-controlled study is now in progress.

(b) Older onset pauciarticular JCA

This group is clinically and genetically heterogenous and includes arthritis associated with psoriasis and inflammatory bowel disease. Juvenile ankylosing spondylitis is another subgroup, affecting mainly boys in their first decade and causing asymmetrical large joint involvement in the lower limbs, and enthesopathy. Many are positive for HLA B27. A typical pattern of joint involvement might be a hip, the tarsal and knee joints. Our 15 year follow-up shows that back involvement occurs in approximately 60% of these children after, but not usually before, adolescence. Apart from NSAIDs, sulphasalazine may be effective.[6]

Polyarticular JCA

Polyarticular JCA is usually obvious with five or more joints becoming affected more or less symmetrically in the first 3–6 months. Children are often referred to a specialist sooner rather than later. However, a small proportion with so-called 'dry arthritis' do not have active synovitis but gradually develop contractures which are often missed until the later stages when deformities are evident. Loss of function or range of movement at a joint in the absence of pain and swelling should act as a reminder of this condition.

Polyarticular JCA is further subdivided according to whether it is rheumatoid factor (RF) negative or positive. The majority of children are negative for RF of IgG and other classes of immunoglobulin. RF positive JCA has a similar clinical picture to adult rheumatoid arthritis (RA). Remission may occur in about 50% of all polyarticular cases but the rate is certainly not as high as in the pauciarticular group. Anti-malarial treatment should be given early in both RF positive and negative cases, using hydroxy-chloroquine in doses of up to 6.5 mg/kg daily, to limit disease progression. If a 6 month trial fails, gold therapy is likely to be effective for RF positive arthritis, as in adult RA. Low dose methotrexate is effective in both types. Regular specialist supervision is essential to prevent and minimise complications, but primary care physicians and paediatricians have important roles in monitoring drug therapy and development, supervising physiotherapy and helping the child and family to cope.

Systemic onset JCA

Systemic onset JCA usually begins before the age of 5 yrs but can occur throughout childhood. It presents with a characteristic high fever, a salmon pink or red maculopapular rash, myalgia, lymphadenopathy and enlargement of the liver and spleen. Arthritis affects the knees, wrists, ankles and neck followed by other joints.[4,5] It has many mimics, such as neuroblastoma, leukaemia, infections and connective tissue diseases, so systemic JCA is partly a diagnosis by exclusion.

Physiotherapy, splinting and NSAIDs to control pain, inflammation and fever are all important in management. Daily or alternate day steroids are very effective in severe disease but, because of long-term side effects on metabolism, growth and bone density, methotrexate is currently under study. Other second line drugs are either disappointing or even dangerous during exacerbations of systemic disease.

Systemic onset JCA is the most severe form of JCA, recurrent episodes of systemic disease occuring in half the cases and progressive arthritis in about a third. Intercurrent infection can trigger a catastrophic exacerbation of disease with liver failure and coagulopathy, whilst amyloidosis occurs in about 10%.[7,8] Both of these complications have an associated mortality.

Hospital and community management of JCA

To support and satisfy the needs of a child with a chronic disease, a multidisciplinary team approach is essential. The hospital specialist will have devised a long term programme of care to prevent or minimise growth deformities, contractures and complications of drug treatment. This programme needs to be discussed with the local paediatrician and family doctor so that they are confident to fulfil their own agreed roles. These might include the monitoring of drug therapy and the coordination of local services to provide satisfactory education and family support. Children with JCA need regular physiotherapy and exercise monitoring and often develop a good relationship with their physiotherapists. The physiotherapists in the specialist unit and the community are thus well placed to liaise frequently with each other and to communicate with other members of the team.

Rarer connective tissue diseases of childhood

The more unusual problems seen in a specialist paediatric rheumatology unit include the genetic disorders of bone, cartilage and muscle and the inflammatory diseases such as scleroderma, systemic lupus erythematosus (SLE), dermatomyositis and other vasculitides.

Genetic diseases of bony cartilage and muscles

The rare genetic disorders of cartilage and bone tend to present as loss of joint function or as pain and disability. These include epiphyseal dysplasias, Ehlers-Danlos syndrome and osteogenesis imperfecta. Such patients are usually referred to a specialist and the diagnosis is often made on physical appearance and X-ray, although some cases also need tissue biopsies. Problems like mucopolysaccharidoses and mucolipidoses are more complicated and require metabolic investigation at specialist centres. Congenital neuromuscular disorders may also present as rheumatology problems and often need referral on to a neuromuscular unit. All these cases need the full support of a team approach to care and in addition there may be the need for genetic counselling.

Connective tissue diseases

Most cases of juvenile scleroderma are of the localised type which tends to have a self-limiting natural history, although considerable deformities can result. The rarer linear type can cause severe growth deformities of subcutaneous tissue, underlying muscle and bone. Therapy of these conditions is under evaluation and anecdotal reports suggest that D-penicillamine in doses of up to 10mg/kg/day may accelerate resolution although, as in adults, it does not improve systemic sclerosis.

Childhood SLE is clinically the same as the adult disease and so is the treatment. The onset of nephritis can be very rapid so requent monitoring of urine, blood pressure and serum electrolytes by the primary care physician is essential. Dermatomyositis is often a 'one-hit' disease, usually with muscle tenderness and a high serum creatine phosphokinase. The dramatic deterioration in muscle strength can be life threatening especially if it involves the intercostal and palatal muscles. Early high dose steroid treatment is effective but it needs to be given daily, not on alternate days, and dose reductions must be slow. Other immunosuppressive agents, such as azathioprine and cyclosporin A, have proved effective.

SLE, other vasculitides and dermatomyositis sometimes present insidiously in childhood so the main features might be just general malaise, poor appetite, irritability or marked behavioural change. The range of childhood vasculitides also includes polyarteritis nodosa, Kawasaki disease (the mucocutaneous lymph node syndrome), Henoch-Schonlein purpura and post-streptococcal cutaneous vasculitis which is often mistakenly diagnosed as arthritis because of its peri-articular lesions. The onset of a characteristic rash should alert to the possibility of vasculitis and a raised ESR will suggest an inflammatory process whilst a blood count may show the normochromic normocytic anaemia of chronic disease. Anti-neutrophil cytoplasmic antibodies may be positive in Wegener's granulomatosis and microscopic polyarteritis. Rapid referral and close communication are vital for the early diagnosis and management of these conditions.

Steroid treatment, with pulsed intravenous cyclophosphamide in severe cases, is effective in the management of most polyarteritides. Intravenous gammaglobulin is also particularly effective in Kawasaki disease where it prevents coronary artery aneurysms. Clinical trials are in progress to see whether it may also be effective in other types of vasculitis.

Conclusion

Many aches and pains of childhood are mild and self-limiting. Others are more persistent and benefit from confirmation of the diagnosis by a specialist, after which there is often recovery with rest and physiotherapy. Juvenile chronic arthritides are distressing and need a carefully planned programme of care to allow the affected child and family as full and as normal a life as possible. This is best achieved by a multidisciplinary approach perhaps involving paediatric rheumatologist, paediatrician, primary care physician and their combined physiotherapy and rehabilitation resources. Such principles also apply to the rarer connective tissue disorders where there is the same need to monitor growth and to supervise potentially toxic and complex drug treatments. These therapies, in turn, are the subject of wide ranging clinical trials.

References

1. Prieur AM, Le Gall E, Karman F, Edan C, Lasserre O, Goujard J. Epidemiological survey of juvenile chronic arthritis in France. Comparison of data obtained from two different regions. *Clin Exp Rheumatol* 1987; **5**: 217–23.
2. Towner SR, Michet CJ, O'Fallon WM, Nelson A. The epidemiology of juvenile arthritis in Rochester Minnesota 1960–79. *Arthritis Rheum* 1983; **26**: 1208–13.
3. Ansell BM, Rudge S, Schaller JG. *A colour atlas of paediatric rheumatology*. London: Wolfe, 1991.
4. Prieur AM, Ansell BM, Bardfield R et al. Is onset type evaluation during the first 3 months of disease satisfactory for defining the subgroups of juvenile chronic arthritis? A EULAR co-operative study (1983–1986). *Clin Exp Rheumatol* 1990; **8**: 321–5.
5. Cassidy JT, Levinson JE, Brewer EJ. The development of classification criteria for children with juvenile rheumatoid arthritis. *Bull Rheum Dis* 1989; **38**: 1–7.
6. Ansell BM, Hall MA, Loftus JK, Woo P et al. A multicentre pilot study of sulphasalazine in juvenile chronic arthritis. *Clin Exp Rheumatol* 1991; **9**: 201–3.
7. Stoeber E. Progression of juvenile chronic arthritis. *Eur J Pediatr* 1981; **135**: 225–8.
8. David J, Vouyiouka O, Ansell BM, Hall A, Woo P. Amyloidosis in juvenile chronic arthritis: a morbidity and mortality study. *Clin Exp Rheumatol* 1993; **11**: 85–90.

5 | Back pain: concepts in pathogenesis

Malcolm IV Jayson
Rheumatic Diseases Centre, University of Manchester

Back pain is one of the commonest disorders affecting our society. The peak incidence occurs in the most productive years and it is the commonest cause of loss of work in those under the age of 45 years.[1] Incidence and prevalence have increased so greatly that loss of work due to back pain has risen by 300% since 1940 whereas that due to illness as a whole has increased by only 50%. In the UK it is responsible for some 60 million working days lost per annum and 13% of all sickness incapacity. The annual cost to our society has been estimated at £3,000 million. In the United States back injuries constitute 19% of all workers' compensation claims and 41% of total injury costs.[2]

Chronic back pain and disability arise for a number of reasons, and each case requires detailed assessment to identify remediable causes. The situation with chronic back pain is quite different from the acute problems which usually resolve fairly rapidly with conservative therapy. Careful assessment is certainly necessary to exclude chronic conditions such as ankylosing spondylitis or herniated intervertebral discs for which useful therapeutic strategies are available. Unfortunately, there is also a large residue of patients with severe chronic back pain for whom no entirely satisfactory treatment can be offered. Some will have undergone one or more previous spinal operations and will be left with varying degrees of permanent disability. Such cases might have instability or degenerative disease of the spine, central or foraminal stenoses, microfractures or a history of oil-based contrast materials used for myelography. Chronic symptoms and disability may cause, and also be aggravated by, psychological and emotional disturbance. It seems likely that a greater understanding of pathogenesis might lead to more successful management of these very difficult cases.

This chapter describes a role for vascular damage, fibrosis and chronic inflammation as a cause of symptoms and disability. Treatment aimed at preventing and correcting such vascular damage may offer a new and effective therapeutic approach.

Clinical Background

The traditional classification of back and spinal pain separates
mechanical problems from inflammatory disorders such as ankylosing spondylitis. Mechanical causes are by far the most common but
objective evidence of mechanical damage often correlates poorly
with symptoms. Whilst there is some relationship between back
pain and radiological change,[3] it is striking how some patients with
trivial degenerative disease have severe and persistent pain whereas
others with advanced damage on X-ray may be symptom free. The
clinical pattern of mechanical back pain is often one of fluctuating
symptoms, an acute episode usually remitting rapidly after which
there may well be a symptom free interlude or only minor problems
until the next acute episode. However, degenerative changes in the
spine do not fluctuate, so mechanical damage is not an adequate
explanation for symptoms in many patients, indicating that other
factors must also play an important role.

Many back pain sufferers complain of marked stiffness on
waking, on resting and when sitting still in a chair. This contrasts
with the anticipated pattern of a mechanical problem in which pain
and stiffness should be relieved by rest and aggravated by exercise.
It is more suggestive of vascular and chronic inflammatory
processes and, indeed, there is evidence of these. Radiculograms
in patients with disc prolapse often show nerve root swelling,
indicating the presence of oedema, and dilated veins may
also be obvious in spinal stenosis where the nerve roots are
crowded. At surgery an erythematous layer may be found covering
the nerve roots and this is most marked when disc rupture is
complete to the outer border of the annulus fibrosus. This
increased vascularity can be demonstrated by intravenous
enhanced CAT and MRI scanning as an area of enhancement at the
edge of the prolapse.[4] In spines where there has been no previous
surgical intervention this erythematous layer, often called 'vascular
granulation tissue', consists of dilated blood vessels and fibrosis but
without active inflammation.

During laminectomy under local anaesthetic, sciatic pain occurs
normal nerve roots. Histologically the damaged roots may
show changes similar to those in spinal stenosis[5] with perineu-
rial hyperplasia and chronic inflammatory cell infiltration.
Multiple adhesions are also often found round damaged nerve
roots and these secondary changes may also contribute towards
symptoms.

Arachnoiditis and peridural fibrosis

Chronic inflammation and scarring can occur within the dural sheath (arachnoiditis) and in the surrounding tissues (peridural fibrosis), compressing and distorting nerve roots. Many patients with these findings suffer severe back and referred pain, perhaps because of direct pressure effects but also possibly because of loss of afferent neurones within the nerve roots. To investigate these mechanisms further we looked at intervertebral foramina from cadaveric specimens, examining the relationship between degenerative disease, epidural venous plexus compression and venous obstruction, perineural fibrosis, intraneural fibrosis and neuronal atrophy.[6] Prolapsed discs and osteophytes rarely seemed to compress nerve roots directly but there was frequent evidence of venous compression which correlated with the extent of disc degeneration and herniation. Venous compression was associated with dilatation of non-compressed veins in the intervertebral foramina and venous thromboses. Changes in blood vessels within the perineural fibrotic tissue included damage to endothelial cells with basement membrane thickening, platelet adhesion and, in some cases, intravascular fibrin deposition and fibrosis. The amount of venous dilatation correlated with the development of perineural fibrosis and in the nerve roots affected in this way there was loss of myelinated neurones. These findings are similar to those in other conditions, such as lipodermatosclerosis, in which venous obstruction also leads to vascular injury and fibrosis. They therefore suggest that mechanical changes in the spine can lead to vascular damage with venous obstruction, causing tissue ischaemia and stimulating fibrosis which in turn damages nerve roots.

Arachnoiditis, which leads to severe fibrosis, used to be caused mainly by infection but it is now seen most frequently after spinal surgery and oil-based contrast myelography. Early inflammation of the pia and arachnoid leads to fibroblast proliferation and fibrin adhesions around nerve roots. This progresses to end stage adhesive arachnoiditis with dense collagen encapsulating nerve roots which become hypoaemic and undergo extensive atrophy.

In biopsy specimens, which we examined from patients with epidural fibrosis undergoing repeat surgery to remove extensive scar tissue, there was gross proliferating collagenous tissue with inflammatory cell infiltrates and dilated veins. On polarised light microscopy the chronic inflammatory cell infiltrates were concentrated around birefringent deposits of cotton fragments.[7] These findings suggest that retained cotton debris from swabs and patties used at surgery was responsible for the subsequent development of excessive scar tissue. In other specimens we found radio-opaque liquid droplets which we identified as retained medium from previous oil-based myelography.

These observations indicate that vascular damage and fibrosis are common in many mechanical back problems. In spines in which there has been no previous intervention there is no evidence of an inflammatory element. However, when there has been previous intervention, usually surgery or oil-based myelography, focal accumulations of chronic inflammatory cells may be seen which might account for the more severe problems in such cases.

Studies of the fibrinolytic system

After tissue injury fibrinogen polymerises to form fibrin which is deposited to form clot. There is also a temporary decrease in fibrinolysis which gradually returns to normal over a few weeks so that fibrin is eventually cleared and tissues return to normal. The fibrinolytic enzyme system is a complex cascade of reactions in which tissue plasminogen activator catalyses the conversion of plasminogen to plasmin. This clears fibrin to form fibrin degradation products. There are several inhibitors of this system including tissue plasminogen activator inhibitor which, in excess, will lead to defective fibrinolytic activity. A persistent reduction in fibrinolytic activity, with failure to clear fibrin, might interfere with oxygen and nutrient supplies to tissues and thus cause chronic tissue damage. This mechanism is of interest in that smoking, which produces a defect in the thrombolytic system, is also associated with back pain, and in pain-free individuals it is a risk factor for the subsequent development of back problems.[8]

In our own studies of patients with chronic back pain we found decreased fibrinolytic activity due to an excess of tissue plasminogen activator inhibitor. Not all patients showed this change, neither did it correlate with individual clinical or imaging features but it was much more frequent in those with the worst back problems and this applied across diagnostic groups. When we looked at advanced radiological features of lumbar spondylosis and compared patients with and without chronic back pain, the defect seemed a better marker for the presence of pain than radiological changes alone. Changes were most marked in patients with the worst back problems caused by arachnoiditis.[9,10] In prospective studies the fibrinolytic defect correlates with clinical outcome in patients presenting with their first episode of back pain and sciatica[11] and in those undergoing spinal surgery it is an adverse prognostic marker.[12] These findings suggest that, in some cases, a change in fibrinolytic activity might be helpful as an objective marker of the severity of the back problem. It might also act as a secondary pathogenic mechanism, contributing to persistent vascular damage by failing to clear fibrin from damaged blood vessels.

Our observations on the fibrinolytic defect have prompted studies using stanosolol, an anabolic steroid of low virilising potential which stimulates the fibrinolytic system and corrects the defect. In a pilot uncontrolled study we were surprised to find it helpful for back problems where surgery had not been used but not for post-surgical cases.[13] This might suggest that fibrinolytic enhancement is of greatest benefit if given earlier rather than later. We are therefore undertaking prospective studies to see if fibrinolytic enhancement can prevent post-surgical fibrosis. In addition, because physical activity enhances fibrinolysis, we are also examining the effects of exercise on the fibrinolytic system in these patients in relation to clinical outcome.

Sympathetic dysfunction syndrome

Sympathetic dysfunction has been suggested as a cause of chronic pain and lower limb symptoms in patients with disc prolapse, spinal surgery, oil-based myelography and traumatic myelopathy.[14,15] Many of these patients describe chronic burning lower extremity pain often associated with allodyna and hyperpathia. Neurological examination and imaging provide no evidence of radicular damage. Criteria for assessing this syndrome have not been established and sympathectomy has been used rather indiscriminately with confusing results. Using thermography and quantified sweat measurements in patients with chronic unilateral lower limb pain referred from the lumbar spine we have demonstrated evidence of sympathetic overactivity correlating with the distribution of symptoms. In such patients treated by local sympathetic block, preliminary results show a transient relief of pain with a return of thermographic appearances and peripheral autonomic potential to normal. Sympathetic nervous system overactivity therefore seems to play an important role in the pathogenesis of pain in this group of patients so the case for surgical sympathectomy is now being evaluated in more detail.

Conclusions

We now believe that vascular damage in various forms plays an important role in the pathogenesis of many chronic mechanical back problems. An understanding of the basic pathology should lead to specific forms of treatment which, hopefully, will produce significant advances in management of this seemingly intractable problem.

Acknowledgments

I wish to thank Drs Therese Brammah, R Cooper, AJ Freemont, R Gush, K Hadidy, Judith Hoyland, Anita Keegan, P Klimiuk, R Million, W Mitchell, Gillian Pountain, Miss Karen Illingworth and Miss Carol Sweet, all of whom have participated in this research programme.

References

1. Carey TS. Occupational back pain: issues in prevention and treatment. *Baillière's Clin Rheumatol* 1989; **3**: 143–56.
2. Spengler DM, Bigos SJ, Martin NA, Zeh J, Fisher L, Nachemson A. Back injuries in industry: a retrospective study. 1. Overview and cost analysis. *Spine* 1986; **11**: 241–5.
3. Lawrence JS. *Rheumatism in populations*. London: Heinemann, 1977.
4. Firooznia H, Kricheff II, Rafii M, Golimbu C. Lumbar spine after surgery: examination with contrast enhanced CT. *Radiology* 1987; **163**: 221–6.
5. Watanabe R, Parke WW. The vascular and neural pathology of lumbosacral spinal stenosis. *J Neurosurg* 1986; **64**: 64–70.
6. Hoyland JA, Freemont AJ, Jayson MIV. Intervertebral foramen venous obstruction: a cause of periradicular fibrosis? *Spine* 1989; **14**: 558–68.
7. Hoyland JA, Freemont AJ, Denton J, Thomas AMC, McMillan JJ, Jayson MIV. Retained surgical swab debris in post-laminectomy arachnoiditis and peridural fibrosis. *J Bone Joint Surg Br* 1988; **70**: 659–62.
8. Battie MC, Bigos SJ, Fisher LD et al. A prospective study of the role of cardiovascular risk factors and fitness in industrial back pain complaints. *Spine* 1989; **14**: 141–7.
9. Pountain GD, Keegan AL, Jayson MIV. Impaired fibrinolytic activity in defined chronic back syndromes. *Spine* 1987; **12**: 83–6.
10. Cooper RG, Mitchell WS, Illingworth KJ, St Clair Forbes W, Gillespie JE, Jayson MIV. The role of epidural fibrosis and defective fibrinolysis in the persistence of post-laminectomy back pain. *Spine* 1991; **16**: 1044–8.
11. Klimiuk PS, Pountain GD, Keegan AL, Jayson MIV. Serial measurements of fibrinolytic activity in acute low back pain and sciatica. *Spine* 1987; **12**: 925–8.
12. Haaland AK, Graver V, Ljunggren AE et al. Fibrinolytic activity as a predictor of outcome of prolapsed intervertebral lumbar disc surgery with respect to background variables: results of a prospective cohort study. *Spine* 1992; **17**: 1022–7.

13. Cooper RG, Mitchell WS, Illingworth KJ, Jayson MIV. Fibrinolytic enhancement with stanozolol fails to improve symptoms and signs in patients with post-surgical back pain. *Scand J Rheumatol* 1991; **20**: 414–8.
14. Carlson DH, Simon H, Wegner W. Bone scanning and diagnosis of reflex sympathetic dystrophy secondary to herniated lumbar discs. *Neurology* 1977; **27**: 791–3.
15. Cremer SA, Maynard F, Davidoff G. The reflex sympathetic dystrophy syndrome associated with traumatic myelopathy: report of five cases. *Pain* 1989; **37**: 187–92.

6 | Sports medicine

Colin P Crosby

Department of Exercise and Sports Medicine, The Garden Hospital, London

The recent Allied Dunbar National Fitness Survey[1] makes it clear that overall activity levels in the UK are considerably lower than are recommended for cardiovascular health. As the medical benefits of exercise become clearer and the risks of inactivity more widely realised[2,3] there is a small but increasing tendency amongst the medical profession to prescribe exercise; this development is welcome. Exercise prescriptions are now advised not only for cardiovascular conditions[4] but also for musculo-skeletal,[5] pulmonary[6] and endocrine disorders.[7] Regular exercise confers psychological benefit[8] and even improves immunological function.[9] Guidelines for safe and effective exercise programmes have been published[10] and these are concerned more with regular, rhythmical activity over a sustained period than with exercise of competitive intensity. As a result of the greater national focus on exercise and keeping fit[2] about 15 million Britons now take part in some form of regular physical activity.

Although the advantages of regular exercise may be quite evident, the problems which may occur should not be underestimated. Over 11 million days of sickness and invalidity benefit are claimed annually as a result of exercise related injury[11] and soft tissue injuries account for at least 7% of all general practice consultations.[12]

Patterns of sports injury

In a recent study association football gave rise to considerably more injuries than any other activity. It was responsible for 8.6 million exercise-related injuries, nearly a third of all those estimated to occur annually. Running, weight training and keep fit each contributed over 2 million injuries and rugby football, squash, badminton and martial arts each contributed about 1.5 million. However, when these figures were related to number of players and frequency of participation, rugby emerged as by far the most dangerous of all sports in the UK. For every 1000 hours' play the number of injuries for rugby was 63.6 compared with 42.2 for soccer, 40.2 for hockey, 27.1 for martial arts, 24.2 for squash, 17.9 for running, 10.4 for horse riding and 9.5 for keep fit. It is interesting that horse riding, long considered one of the most dangerous sports, was six times safer than rugby, but this figure may be unduly reassuring for horse riders as the survey of 16-45 year olds excluded younger riders who might be at relatively greater risk.[11]

Different sports have different injury profiles. Duration events, especially running on unforgiving pavements, entail repeated sub-maximal loading on weight-bearing structures. This can lead to overuse injuries such as plantar fascitis, Achilles tendinitis, stress fractures and synovitis. Vigorous multiple sprint and contact sports tend to produce more direct trauma such as head injuries, lacera-tions and haematomata. Angular momentum of the body with the foot in a fixed position causes rotatory and shear injuries to carti-lage and ligaments. With outdoor events environmental factors give the possibility of hypo- or hyperthermia, sunburn, dehydration and immersion injury. The tri-athlete or fell runner may even face several of these risks in the course of a single race! The level at which an athlete participates may also have an effect on injury profile. At higher levels of competition the rate and severity of injury both increase[11] and pressure to rejoin the sport too soon after injury may be considerable.

Management of sports injuries

Management of sports injuries does not require a knowledge of all sports played in the UK, which now number over one hundred and thirty. It is more useful to have a basic understanding of the mechanical stresses and injury patterns resulting from a few typical activities. These include running, team or individual contact sports and throwing which, in terms of shoulder movement, also takes in the golf swing and the fast bowler's arm action. An appreciation of how high impact activities result in trauma to the back, hip, shin and knee is also vital. A knowledge of anatomy, orthopaedics and rheumatology, especially of joint assessment and injection tech-niques, is essential.[13] The detailed management of each injury is outside the scope of this discussion but there are many excellent texts on the subject.[14,15,16]

Sports injury management often needs a team approach. The physician needs to have a good working relationship with a char-tered physiotherapist, an effective liaison with local coaches and trainers and a familiarity with the popular local sporting activities.

The practitioner and therapist need to reassure the patient and show sympathy at all times since a comparatively minor injury can be devastating to an athlete whose entire social and emotional life may be tied up in sport. The athlete also needs to feel confident in the knowledge and skills of those dealing with his injury.

Successful management of each case needs thoroughness, a clear treatment plan and a realistic acceptance of the outcome in terms of time spent away from the activity which resulted in the injury. For diagnosis, reliance must still be placed on careful clinical assessment with radiology in selected cases. A variety of sophisticated techniques are becoming available, more as research tools but also as ways of permitting greater diagnostic accuracy in elite competitors. These include real-time ultrasonography, radio-isotope scanning, compartment pressure studies, computerised tomography, magnetic resonance imaging and gait analysis. In typical sports injury practice they are rarely appropriate and a practical approach with prompt physiotherapy will lead to a complete return to normal sporting function in the majority of cases. In the past, the minimalist treatment which was usually expected and often given so easily lead to chronic or recurrent injury with loss of fitness, inability to play, time off work and diminished quality of life. A brusque instruction to stop all activity for three weeks, perhaps accompanied by a prescription for an anti-inflammatory drug, not only alienates the patient but also results in loss of fitness, muscle atrophy and frustration.

Care should be taken not to underestimate soft tissue injuries. The painful and bruised inversion injury of the ankle may not show bony damage on X-ray but thorough examination will reveal the torn lateral ligament complex. Proper management may involve surgical repair, true immobilisation and cast-bracing followed by rehabilitation of ligamentous function, muscle strength, ankle proprioception and range of motion. Refractory cases certainly benefit from referral to a specialist sports injury clinic but in practice only 5-10% of all exercise-related injuries actually require surgical intervention. For those cases awaiting an orthopaedic appointment a regular programme of physiotherapy started soon after the injury is likely to be of greater benefit than a long period of inactivity. This programme might include massage, manipulation and exercise with additional electrotherapeutic techniques plus paramedical skills such as osteopathy, chiropody and exercise physiology when needed.

Preventing injury

Doctors dealing with sportsmen and women at any level need to share the corporate responsibility of reducing the chance of injury. The importance of getting fit for sport rather than using sport to get fit should be communicated to the would-be athlete. Pre-exercise screening and fitness testing help to indicate potential problems before they occur. They also set baseline standards of performance against which the effects of training can be measured or whereby recovery can be judged following any future injury. The physician should also emphasise the proper use of protective equipment, whether it be BSI approved helmets for riders, moulded mouth guards for rugby, eye protectors for squash or functioning bindings for skiing. Correct warm-up, stretching exercises and strength training all help to reduce injury[17] and the physician, coach and therapist can all work together to produce appropriate programmes.

Doctors are in a unique position to influence preventive measures at a local level by stating well-founded professional views likely to be respected by athletes, coaches, parents and club administrators. This is especially true if the doctor has involved himself in sporting activities, learnt about them and has been seen to identify with the aims and goals of the athletes and their clubs. At a national level, pressure from physicians can be effective in forcing a change in law to prevent dangerous techniques or manoeuvres and this has already taken place in rugby with considerable reduction in the incidence of serious neck injury.[18]

The pressures on children and other young athletes to perform well can be enormous, often to the detriment of their future musculo-skeletal development.[19] In order to reduce a child's training or competition workload the informed physician may be placed in the difficult position of having to advise a child against what he enjoys doing and is best at, or he may have to defend the child against the ambitions of coaches and parents. In the future these situations may be easier to deal with because of useful changes in regulations, such as agreements on minimum age categories for sports like gymnastics. Weight categories rather than age limits may be appropriate ways of making other sports fairer and safer. In New Zealand this approach has largely removed the size and strength differential found in the age bands for junior rugby.

Sports injury clinics

General practitioners often make excellent sports physicians because of their breadth of interest and experience. The disciplines which are called upon when dealing with the injured athlete are easily illustrated by a few examples: athlete's heart, scrum pox, activity-induced amenorrhoea, hyphaema in the squash player, Osgood-

Schlatter's disease, overtraining syndrome and drug taking. Whilst many primary care physicians will become involved in different aspects of exercise-related injuries, only a few will wish to develop their interest to the extent of setting up their own sports medicine clinics. If they do, detailed recommendations of what is required in an ideal sports injury clinic have been published.[20]

Sports injury clinics are growing rapidly within the private sector but there is little regulation of their personnel, expertise and facilities so standards are still very mixed. The registry of clinics, published by the British Association of Sport and Medicine (BASM), allows the title of 'sports injury clinic' if a medical practitioner and a chartered physiotherapist are both in attendance. The term 'sports physiotherapy clinic' applies if there is only a chartered physiotherapist. The British Olympic Association (BOA) also publishes a sports injury clinic list and the entries have all been visited and accredited. Several regions produce their own local lists and reference can be made to the Sports Council or regional BASM representative. Some useful sources of information are included in the Appendix.

A logical development from the sports injury clinic is the increasing collaboration between the sports physician, local general practitioners and the local sports centre. Suitable programmes can be devised not only for rehabilitation of sports injuries but also for back pain and recovery from cardiac surgery or orthopaedic procedures. Further information on pre-exercise screening, fitness testing, exercise prescription and exercise clinics can be obtained from the Harpenden Sports Centre. For patients attending gym sessions and exercise classes on their doctor's recommendation there may be psychological, emotional and economic benefit as well as physical improvement without undue reliance on drug treatments.

In the United States the larger gyms and sports centres now have their own medical director who works with exercise staff, dieticians and management to produce suitable exercise programmes. Their expertise allows them to satisfy special needs and to give skilled advice to individuals with specific problems. A few centres in the UK are beginning to make such appointments and they represent an ideal opportunity for the physician with an interest in sports medicine to work with motivated and health-conscious people.

Expert advice is certainly needed by a wide range of people keen to involve themselves in exercise. For example, for the sportswomen it may be difficult to decide upon a safe or optimum level of physical activity. There is a fine dividing line between increasing bone density by regular exercise and inducing osteoporosis by the oestrogen deficiency of secondary amenorrhoea which occurs during high intensity training. The aerobics dancer or runner who has recently increased her workload may be at risk of sudden disability from an overuse injury such as a metatarsal stress fracture.[21] Other women who exercise obsessively to disguise eating disorders need to be identified and offered therapy which is more appropriate than over-work in the gym.

The sports physician is bound to come across the increasing prob-lem of drug abuse in sport. So many athletes, professional and ama-teur alike, are prepared to go to any length to improve their performance. Drug abuse is now controlled by strict regulations which can be applied, theoretically at least, to all ages and levels of competition. The value of such regulations is offset by technical difficulties. New substances are continually being produced and new uses are being found for old ones, so regulations tend to be one step behind current drug taking practice. Blood doping and ery-thropoietin injection cannot be exposed by the present method of urine examination and would be extremely difficult to detect even if more invasive blood testing were permitted in the future.

The Sports Council has produced a guide to banned substances and their permitted alternatives[22] and this is an essential reference for athletes and their medical attendants. Greatest care must be exercised in choosing any form of medication for the competitive athlete. A prescription for Benylin linctus may seem entirely reason-able on clinical grounds but its pseudoephedrine content is prohib-ited by the International Olympic Committee. Simple Linctus is permitted.

The way forward

Leisure time is increasing and more people are aware of the need for fitness to maintain good health, so exercise-related injuries are likely to become more common. In the UK an effective system of care for injuries sustained during physical activity is still in its infancy and it seems unlikely, in the present economic climate, that the NHS will fund a sports medicine service as a separate specialty. Initiatives will therefore have to come from other areas such as sporting organisations and the private sector.

Future developments in the field of sports medicine must be underpinned by an effective programme of education. For the doctor this must be at a postgraduate level because the subject is not included in the medical school curriculum. As with any new field, there are many areas of sports medicine which are controversial and in need of further research. The setting up of the new National Sports Medicine Institute (NSMI) is an important step since part of its remit is to work with the Sports Council towards regional and sub-regional sports medicine centres where there will be a commitment to education and research as well as therapy. A diploma in sports medicine is now offered by the Society of Apothecaries of London and by the Royal Colleges of Physicians and Surgeons of Glasgow and Edinburgh. There are now national courses on the subject, some full-time for a year, others part-time of varying length or run as modular distance learning packages. The NSMI and the BASM are always able to give details. The BASM also produces the British Journal of Sports Medicine quarterly and holds regular regional meetings of multi-disciplinary interest for its national membership.

Conclusion

There is increasing emphasis on exercise and physical activity as a way of maintaining good health. The benefits of this may be offset, in some cases, by exercise-related injuries. These need to be treated promptly and expertly to prevent undue long-term disability and disenchantment. Effective treatment needs to be coupled to a process of education and injury prevention at a local and national level. Sports injury services are still in the process of evolution and there is opportunity for interested doctors to become more involved in their future development. As a specialty, sports medicine calls upon a wide range of different disciplines and the team approach to care extends well beyond the clinic into the sports themselves.

References

1. Activity and health research. *Allied Dunbar national fitness survey: a report on activity patterns and fitness levels.* London: The Sports Council and The Health Education Authority, 1992.
2. Fentem PH, Bassey EJ, Turnbull NB. *The new case for exercise.* London: The Sports Council and The Health Education Authority, 1988.
3. The Royal College of Physicians. *Medical aspects of exercise: benefits and risks.* London: The Royal College of Physicians, 1991.
4. Todd IC, Ballantyne D. Antianginal efficacy of exercise training: a comparison with beta blockade. *Br Heart J* 1990; **64**: 14–19.
5. Burry HC. Sports, exercise and arthritis. *Br J Rheumatol* 1987; **26**: 386–8.
6. Bundgaard A. Exercise in the asthmatic. *Sports Med* 1985; **2**: 254–66.

7. Trovati M, Carta Q, Cavalot F et al. Influence of physical training on blood glucose control, glucose tolerance, insulin secretion and insulin action in non-insulin dependent diabetic patients. *Diabetes Care* 1984; **7**: 416–20.

8. Martinsen EW. Physical fitness, anxiety and depression. *Br J Hosp Med* 1990; **43**: 194–9.

9. Sharp NC, Koutedakis Y. Sport and the overtraining syndrome: immunological aspects. *Br Med Bull* 1992; **48**: 3, 518–33.

10. Health Education Council. *Exercise: why bother?* London: The Sports Council, 1986.

11. Nicholl JP, Coleman P, Williams BT. *A national study of the epidemiology of exercise-related injury and illness.* A report to the Sports Council. Sheffield: University of Sheffield Medical School, 1991.

12. Moll H. *Rheumatology in clinical practice.* London: Blackwell Scientific, 1987: 499.

13. Cyriax J. *Textbook of Orthopaedic Medicine. 8th edn.* London: Baillière Tindall, 1982.

14. Read M, Wade P. *Sports injuries: a unique guide to self-diagnosis and rehabilitation.* London: Brelisch and Foss, 1989.

15. Hutson MA. *Sports injuries: recognition and management.* Oxford: Oxford University Press, 1990.

16. Pederson L, Renstrom P. *Sports injuries: their prevention and treatment.* London: Martin Dunitz, 1986.

17. Cahill BR, Griffith EH. Effect of preseason conditioning on the incidence and severity of high school football knee injuries. *Am J Sports Med* 1987; **6**: 180–4.

18. Burry HC, Calcinai CJ. The need to make rugby safer. *Br Med J* 1988; **296**: 149–50.

19. Stulberg SG, Cordell LD, Harris WH et al. Unrecognised childhood hip disease: a main cause of idiopathic osteoarthritis of the hip. In: *The hip: Proceedings of the third open scientific meeting of the hip society.* St. Louis: Mosby, 1975; **3**: 212–8.

20. Read M. What to look for at a sports injury clinic. *Coaching Focus* No 11, National Coaching Foundation, 1989.

21. Krolner B, Toft B, Nielson SP, Tondevold E. Physical exercise as prophylaxis against involutional vertebral bone loss: a controlled trial. *Clin Sci* 1983; **64**: 541–6.

22. The Sports Council. *Drugs in sport: a comprehensive guide to the responsible use of drugs in sport, detailing banned and permitted products.* London: Media Medica, 1991.

Appendix: Useful addresses for the sports physician

Active Health Sports Medicine Clinics
Harpenden Sports Centre
Rothamsted Park, Leyton Road
Harpenden, Herts, AL5 2HU
Tel: 0582 841158

Association of Chartered Physiotherapists in Sports Medicine
Honorary secretary: Miss J Wright
C/o Nottingham School of Physiotherapy
Hucknall Road
Nottingham NG5 1PG
Tel: 0602 627681

British Association of Sport and Medicine
Honorary secretary: Mr Roger Hackney
15 Northfield Road, Chilwell, Notts
Tel: 071 251 0583

British Olympic Association
Church Row, Wandsworth Plain
London SW19 1ES
Tel: 081 871 2677

National Sports Medicine Institute
Medical Collage of St Bartholomew's Hospital
Charterhouse Square
London EC1M 6BQ
Tel: 071 251 0583

The Sports Council
16 Upper Woburn Place
London WC1H 0QP
Tel: 071 388 1277

7 | Primary care management of rheumatoid disease

John Dickson
Primary Care Rheumatology Society, Northallerton, North Yorkshire

Rheumatic complaints account for about 8% of a general practice work load so that in a practice of 2000 patients a GP will deal with perhaps 10 such problems each week. In this group of new and follow-up cases, non-articular rheumatism, back problems and arthritis will each constitute one third of the patients. Of those presenting with a new rheumatic episode the proportions are slightly different in that half will have non-articular rheumatism, a quarter will have back pain and a quarter will have arthritis.[1]

For the majority of patients who present with a new rheumatic complaint, effective management is possible on history and examination without need for laboratory tests or X-rays. A personal knowledge of the patient helps to put symptoms into perspective especially when there are emotional or financial problems at home. Sometimes, an exact diagnosis is not possible so the problem needs to be expressed in terms of a provisional formula for action. If it falls into the 'unknown but not serious' category it can be dealt with by an initial prescription for rest, analgesics and local measures. Any clinical uncertainty, which has to be tolerated whilst giving expedient treatment, can then be overcome by timely review of the patient, often after a few days.

Occasionally there may be need for more vigorous investigation. There might be lack of expected improvement over 2–3 weeks, evidence of systemic disturbance with continued weight loss and raised ESR or suspicion of an underlying systemic disease such as hypothyroidism, neoplasia or Parkinson's disease.

In the present day, the aims of primary care rheumatology must be to provide quality care at a local level. There is also the need to identify accurately the small number of highly selected patients who require specialist referral and hospital care. Inappropriate hospital referral is not only inconvenient for both the patient and the specialist, it is also considerably more expensive than primary care and uses scarce resources which need to be protected. For these reasons, general practitioners and local specialists need to agree upon plans of care for the efficient management of rheumatic diseases. Rheumatoid arthritis is a good model.

Diagnosis and assessment

The Primary Care Rheumatology Society (PCRS) was founded in 1987 to promote education and research in general practice rheumatology. Developing protocols is never easy but one of our early projects was to produce guidelines for the diagnosis and management of rheumatoid arthritis. We decided, in collaboration with our consultant colleagues, that a GP should feel confident with the diagnosis of rheumatoid arthritis if there is persistent symmetrical joint inflammation of greater that eight weeks' duration, early morning stiffness, a positive rheumatoid factor and the absence of clinical pointers to other diseases. Additional support is given to the diagnosis if the ESR is greater than 35, if the plasma viscosity is elevated or if there are erosions on X-ray. The pointers to an alternative diagnosis included skin or nail abnormalities, a history of inflammatory bowel disease, urinary problems or discharge, an ESR greater than 75, a negative rheumatoid factor and a positive antinuclear factor.

In general practice a formal systematic approach to the assessment of rheumatoid arthritis is sometimes necessary but in most cases the specialist methods are unduly complex and time consuming. They tend to give way to a more rapid, functional method of person assessment based on prior knowledge of the patient and often a long-standing relationship. At the time of diagnosis the GP is already likely to know a lot about the patient with rheumatoid arthritis. He will have visited the house and will know the patient's commitments, life style, personal values and expectations. Against this background it is often easy to detect the changes in mental and emotional state, social circumstances and ability to cope caused by the additional burden of disease. Mobility and disability can be assessed repeatedly by observing the patient performing activities around the home and by asking whether there are problems with washing, dressing, cooking or work. This information can be easily recorded in the case notes or computerised records using a simple assessment scale[2] or a notation specific to the practice. Pain, feelings of well-being, morale, levels of physical activity, ability to cope and quality of life can all be scored subjectively on a visual analogue scale if this is thought helpful.

Second line drug therapy

The decision to refer a case for an expert opinion is based on a variety of factors and sometimes it is simply because the patient or relatives request it. However, referral is often coupled to the possible need for second line drugs and in some cases this will be sooner rather than later. Some cases may be young, their disease may have presented acutely or may show an aggressive course early on. There may be loss of function or a pressing need to preserve function, for example in the hands of an artist or pianist. Others will be elderly and a small reduction in function will have a disproportionately large effect on their ability to live alone. In any case it may be prudent to refer a case if there is persistent polysynovitis for 12· weeks or more.

A major question a GP must ask himself is whether he wishes to use second line drug therapy for rheumatoid arthritis without considering referral to a specialist. A preparedness to do this implies that he is also willing to provide for all other aspects of care needed by such a case. For example he should understand the process of synovitis and joint damage and the role and limitations of non-steroidal anti-inflammatory drugs (NSAIDs) when used alone. He should have access to physiotherapy, occupational therapy and other services, such as chiropody, psychology and appliances. The risks and benefits of second line drugs should be explained to the patient and facilities should be satisfactory for monitoring both blood and urine. There should also be a system to identify and recall defaulters. In practice, if a policy for starting second line therapies has been agreed with the local rheumatologist, and if communications are good, a second line drug could well be started by a GP pending the consultant opinion, perhaps a few months later. If the patient tolerates this treatment the visit to the specialist might then concentrate on evaluating its clinical benefit and thus formulating a policy for the next stage of therapy.

The aim of second line drugs is to suppress the rheumatoid disease process, to reduce joint damage and to preserve function. Their benefit has been confirmed in the short term over 1–2 years but there is unfortunately little evidence that they improve long-term outcome over 15–25 years.[3] In our discussions at the PCRS we decided that second line drugs should be used for persistent disease activity of more than nine months' duration despite treatment with a number of NSAIDs. The indicators of persistent disease activity included: morning stiffness lasting 60 minutes or more, three or more swollen and tender joints, an ESR of 30 or more and joint erosions on X-ray. These guidelines may be satisfactory for the majority of milder cases seen in general practice but there will clearly be cases where second line drugs will need to be started sooner than nine months and indeed there is now a trend towards much earlier use of these agents.[4] Patients with aggressive and disabling disease certainly do benefit from early referral to a rheumatologist, perhaps even at the point of diagnosis, and a large percentage of these cases will be started on second line treatment soon afterwards.

It is difficult to formulate a rigid protocol for starting second line drug therapy so the decision still needs to be made on an individual basis.[5] It is perhaps unfortunate that the most powerful second line drugs are also potentially the most toxic. Whilst penicillamine and intramuscular gold may produce dramatic improvement in joint function there is also the possibility that their side effects may make an ill patient feel even worse. They are therefore best used in aggressive disease where the need to produce rapid remission justifies the risk of the high incidence of side effects. Some of these cases may also need steroid treatment and they certainly need to be under the supervision of a rheumatologist. For disease with a slower tempo enteric coated sulphasalazine can be tried first. Nausea and dizziness may be minimised by starting at a dose of 500 mg once daily and increasing by increments of 500 mg every 10 days or so to a maintenance dose of 1 gm twice daily. Methotrexate and azathioprine have tended to be used when other second line drugs are not tolerated or ineffective, but methotrexate is now being used more widely and has a relatively rapid onset of action. Antimalarials are relatively weak and apart from having the avoidable problem of ocular toxicity tend to be better tolerated than other agents so they are useful for mild disease. Oral gold, although less toxic than intramuscular gold, is less effective.[5,6]

Although monitoring schedules are widely recommended for second line drugs[6] it is just as well to have a locally agreed protocol which can also serve as a basis for audit of care. Monitoring the safety of such drugs in general practice has become more straightforward with the advent of computerised records and recalling systems and with the involvement of the practice nurse in chronic disease management. For patients on gold, penicillamine and immunosuppressants, the results of regular blood and urine tests can be entered into a co-operation card and shown at any clinic visit. Similarly, results of any blood tests requested by the GP or the hospital specialist can be copied to both by arrangement with the local laboratory. Patients should also be told to attend for review at any time if symptoms such as rash, bruising or acute infection suggest an adverse effect of treatment.

The efficacy of second line drugs should be assessed perhaps every four to six weeks initially, then every three to four months thereafter. Their onset of action is sometimes disappointingly slow for the patient so it may be six months before a firm decision is made to either continue or stop treatment. During this time an overall assessment of well-being may be a guide to whether a chosen drug has promise. A more formal assessment can include measurement of pain on a visual analogue scale, duration of early morning stiffness, the number of joints actively involved and the ESR or plasma viscosity. Progress and problems should also be discussed with other members of the team, such as the nurse, physiotherapist and occupational therapist, and the patient should be involved in these meetings.

Withdrawing second line treatments, as with starting them, presents a variety of dilemmas, unless adverse effects are the reason for withdrawal, so if care is being shared with the local specialist he should be consulted before definite action is taken. A drug which seems relatively ineffective may still be doing some good by stabilising a downhill clinical course but without producing the clear remission which had been hoped for. Yet if a further second line drug is to be tried the initial choice should be stopped if possible, partly because the benefit of dual therapy is unproven[5] and partly to avoid the problems of combined toxicity. There may then be a period of weeks or months during which the protection offered by one drug may be lost whilst the benefit of the other is awaited and unproven. During this time the patient, frustrated by symptoms and disability, is likely to need a lot of support and encouragement. Finally, for the patient in remission who would like to stop a second line drug there is the problem of knowing whether this will result in an exacerbation of disease. The best course of action is to discuss the position as frankly as possible with the patient and to reduce the drug to the lowest possible therapeutic dose for six months before considering the subject again. Many patients will ultimately decide for themselves and stop treatment.

Supporting the patient

The familiarity and trust shared between the patient and the primary health care team are important in maintaining morale when symptoms of disease become obtrusive. In some cases support needs to be offered in a neutral way by simply spending time with the patient and showing interest and warmth. This allows good communication between doctor and patient without implying undue medical dependence or interfering with the patient's feelings of personal responsibility. For some patients, who are able to attend the practice without too much difficulty, sessions with the practice nurse may help to resolve emotional and personal difficulties without recourse to antidepressants or other drug treatments. For more disabled cases, regular home visits by the doctor benefit the carers as well as the patient, in addition to giving an opportunity to assess therapy.

Many patients, realistic as they are about the nature of their chronic disease, like to feel that there is light at the end of their particular tunnel. This hope, and a positive effect on morale, can be nurtured by maintaining a feeling of momentum in the plan of care. In some cases this will be achieved by a readiness to experiment with different NSAIDs to relieve pain and stiffness. Other patients will benefit from courses of physiotherapy, hydrotherapy, splinting or steroid injections into selected joints.[7,8] A domiciliary occupational therapist can advise on useful aids and adaptation of the home whilst a social worker can explore the range of permitted financial allowances. In some cases, where mobility has declined because of accident, depression or recent viral illness, a brief admission to hospital may restore sufficient function for independent life at home again. An occasional period of respite care in a local community hospital may also relieve the dutiful family and thus help to keep the patient in the community for longer.

Patients have a particular need for support when making decisions which affect their self esteem and long-term life style. This occurs when prolonged absence from work leads to issues like redundancy, retraining and early retirement. The GP is also often involved in the decision to move house, especially when a case for priority treatment has to be presented to the local housing authorities. Even so, the apparent benefit from the improved amenities of rehousing may be so offset by severance from carers, neighbours, friends and their GP that many patients ultimately prefer to stay where they are known.

Contracts

The contracting process for specific diseases continues to evolve. District purchasers and budget holding GPs are still buying services in general terms but it seems likely that they will soon become more specific. Any developments must be made to work to the advantage of the patient, opening up resources and facilitating specialist involvement when needed. For example, satisfactory contracts for prompt orthopaedic surgery for rheumatoid patients would represent a major advance in care. Apart from increasing quality of life, timely joint surgery would also reduce the cost of care in the community.

Inevitably, all services should be used as cost-effectively as possible and if GPs gain open access to more hospital-based facilities they will still need to learn how to use them with discretion. A valuable alternative would be the greater development of community physiotherapy and occupational therapy services which would benefit not only patients with rheumatoid disease but also those with other disabling diseases. The level of communication between the GP, the patient and the rheumatology team needs to develop to keep pace with the complexities of modern management. This might be achieved by community-based specialist nurses or therapists who would help to support patients at home and also provide the necessary liaison between the other members of the team providing care.

Conclusion

A spectrum of rheumatic diseases presents to general practice and in many cases can be diagnosed with minimum investigation and treated symptomatically. The more complex conditions require a greater appreciation of rheumatology and thus the Primary Care Rheumatology Society was founded to promote general practice education and research within the subject.

For rheumatoid arthritis it is helpful for GPs and their local rheumatologist to agree guidelines for care so that management can be successful and cost-effective. Accurate diagnosis, prompt initial management, appropriate referral for second line therapy and monitoring of such therapy can all be described in local protocols. The exact choice and timing of such second line drugs remain subjects for debate.

With good communication each member of the therapeutic team can make a useful contribution to patient care. A strength of the GP is his supportive relationship throughout a chronic illness and his ability to coordinate the many elements of care necessary to optimise quality of life for the patient with rheumatoid arthritis. New contractual arrangements create an opportunity for new ways of providing care and for a greater proportion of this to be provided in the community.

References

1. Knox JDE. Rheumatic diseases: a general practitioner's view. *Baillière's Clin Rheumatol* 1987; **1**: 601–22.
2. Wills J. Simple scale for assessing level of dependency of patients in general practice. *Br Med J* 1986; **292**: 1639–40.
3. Pincus T. Rheumatoid arthritis: disappointing long term outcomes despite successful clinical trials. *J Clin Epidemiol* 1988; **41**: 1037–41.
4. Spector TD, Thompson PW, Evans SJW, Scott DL. Are slow-acting antirheumatic drugs being given earlier in rheumatoid arthritis? *Br J Rheumatol* 1988; **27**: 498–9.
5. Porter DR, Sturrock RD. Medical management of rheumatoid arthritis. *Br Med J* 1993; **307**: 425–8.
6. Anon. Slow-acting antirheumatic drugs. *Drug Ther Bull* 1993; **31**: 17–20.
7. Clarke AK. Injection of joints and periarticular tissues. *This volume*, Ch 11.
8. Chamberlain MA. Rehabilitation of rheumatic diseases. *This volume*, Ch 12.

8 | Systemic lupus erythematosus

Michael L Snaith
Sheffield Centre for Rheumatic Diseases, Sheffield

With a list of about 2000 patients which might generate some 60 cases of back pain annually, a GP might expect to see only one new case of rheumatoid arthritis per year. The other systemic rheumatic diseases, including systemic lupus erythematosus (SLE), Sjögren's syndrome, scleroderma, polymyositis and the various types of vasculitis, are all even less common in primary care. If one takes SLE as an example, the same GP list might have only one case in total, although in some areas of the UK with Afro-Caribbean, Chinese or Asian communities the prevalence is higher.[1] Because of the rarity of these conditions the GP might lack confidence in his ability to make firm diagnoses and he might also be reluctant to become involved in their treatment. Yet he is a vital part of the team approach to such patients and his role may suddenly become of overwhelming importance. There is no substitute for the detailed knowledge and depth of relationship with a patient who, faced with a curious, dangerous or worrying illness will need long-term support and counselling.

The interface between general practice and hospital medicine is constantly changing, presenting new challenges and opportunities. In a large group general practice it might be logical for one partner to support his colleagues by pursuing a special interest in the rheumatic diseases and developing a close liaison with his counterpart, the hospital rheumatologist. His extended case load would then offer sufficient opportunity to gain experience in recognition and detailed case management of rheumatic diseases at an advanced level. The principles which apply to the shared care of rheumatoid arthritis[2] are readily transferable to other rheumatic diseases. Here it is worth looking at SLE as another example of a chronic multisystem disease where a greater share of the general management could be taken over by the GP.

Presentation of SLE

Whilst SLE can develop late in life, most new cases present in women of reproductive age.[3] Arthralgia of small or large joints occurs in over 90% of cases and although it may be quite flitting it is very severe at times.[4] There may be no evidence of synovitis but, if there is, an initial diagnosis of early rheumatoid arthritis might well be suspected. However, SLE rarely presents with a single symptom. Fever and fatigue are almost universal but neither symptom is sufficiently specific to help make a definite diagnosis. Local or generalised lymph node enlargement occurs in well over half the cases but, as it is usually non-tender, it may not be remarked upon initially.

Cutaneous findings occur in 90% of cases of SLE[4] and although the classical photosensitive 'butterfly' rash on the cheeks is very helpful it is only found in 50% of cases. Other rashes may be non-specific and, especially in younger patients, the differential diagnosis tends to include rubella, parvo virus, glandular fever and drug reactions. The presence of cutaneous vasculitis in addition to other presenting symptoms immediately confirms that one is dealing with a significant multisystem disease. It may show as tender infarcts in the nail fold of the fingers or as a blotchy purpuric rash over the palms, soles or tips of the fingers and toes. The marbled appearance of vascular stasis, livedo reticularis, minor variants of which are seen in some normal people in the cold, is a marker for the lupus anticoagulant which is associated with a thrombotic tendency and the antiphospholipid syndrome.[5] Frank purpura usually indicates thrombocytopaenia.

Raynaud's phenomenon is a presenting feature in perhaps 10% of cases of SLE but in the absence of other features of the disease it also raises the possibility of scleroderma or the more localised form of the disease, the CRST syndrome, characterised by calcinosis, Raynaud's phenomenon, sclerodactyly and telangiectasia. Autoantibody testing[5] and clinical course will ultimately indicate the true diagnosis.

Pleuropulmonary involvement is common in SLE.[6] Pleuritic pain with or without pleural effusion occurs in almost half the cases and indicates an immune complex mediated serositis. Isolated episodes of pleurisy, presumed at the time to be infective, are sometimes recalled by patients to have occurred weeks, months or even years before a firm diagnosis is made and suggest an indolent onset and initial course of the disease in such cases. In a young woman such a history raises the additional possibility of pulmonary embolism and infarction which may need to be excluded by ventilation-perfusion scanning.

Cough and breathlessness accompanied by fleeting patchy shadows on chest X-ray may also be caused by SLE but patients need to be referred for further investigation as the differential diagnosis includes infection and other forms of vasculitis such as Wegener's granulomatosis. This multisystem condition is of interest in that it seems more common than previously and milder forms are now being recognised.[7] It also causes dyspnoea and fleeting pulmonary shadowing but in addition there may be nasal involvement which the patient may describe as congestion or sinusitis. In some cases there is a persistent nasal discharge which is bloody at times. Haematuria and proteinuria on dipstick testing indicate the multisystem nature of the disease with renal involvement. Serological testing for antineutrophil cytoplasmic antibodies[5] may help to clarify the diagnosis.

Asthma is not part of the spectrum of SLE but it does occur in polyarteritis nodosa and Churg-Strauss syndrome. These vasculitic conditions tend to occur in older patients and should be suspected if asthma is associated with arthralgia and a rash, particularly if the rash is purpuric. Although these diseases may seem confusing, and the distinction between some of them is made on fine points,[8,9] an appreciation that the patient has a multisystem disease will inevitably lead to further investigation, referral and treatment.

The renal involvement, which occurs in a third to a half of the cases of SLE,[4] is easily misinterpreted before a firm diagnosis has been made. The young woman presenting with fever, malaise and proteinuria might be treated for a presumed urinary infection, the hypertension resulting from the early nephritic process being passed off as a response to anxiety. The subsequent development of a rash might easily be attributed to antibiotic treatment and, indeed, drug rashes are common in SLE, particularly after sulphonamides. In such cases, failure of resolution of what seemed to be a common acute illness soon leads to more detailed investigation in pursuit of an exact diagnosis.

Central nervous system involvement becomes evident in from 14–75% of cases of SLE, the incidence varying according to the diagnostic criteria and investigation methods used.[4,10] It is rarely the initial presentation although some cases come to attention because of emotional lability, psychological disturbance or even psychosis. Some patients describe migrainous attacks, often with visual symptoms predominating over headache.[4] Epilepsy may be disabling, not only because of fits but also because of the necessary ban from driving which interferes with domestic life or prevents continuing employment. Cranial neuropathies may occur and, rarely, spinal cord involvement may suggest an initial diagnosis of demyelination.

Occasional patients who appear to have SLE will turn out to have mixed connective tissue disease (MCTD), a condition showing features of SLE, scleroderma and polymyositis. Most patients have arthralgia or arthritis, sclerodermatous changes in the skin of the hands but not usually to the point of digital ulceration, telangiectasia, and some have an erythematous rash similar to that seen in SLE. Lung disease reminiscent of SLE, with pulmonary shadowing and pleuritic involvement, may be disabling but nephritis is unusual. Cerebral disease is also uncommon in MCTD but there is a curious propensity for cranial nerve palsies to develop on treatment with anti-inflammatory drugs. Although considered by some authorities to be a specific clinical entity, perhaps based on the serological finding of high antibody titres to ribonucleoprotein,[5] the nature of MCTD is often seen to change over prolonged follow up. Patients tend to develop more sclerodermatous features, particularly with lung involvement. Management follows the same general principles used for SLE and more severe cases need steroids and cytotoxic drugs.

Investigation

The initial investigation of suspected SLE is fairly straightforward in that for any multisystem disease each system needs to be evaluated with its own range of basic tests. For mild disease where there is doubt about the possibility of SLE these tests can be arranged by the GP. Results returning within a day or so, taken together with the clinical picture, will help to indicate whether the tempo of disease is slow enough to be dealt with on an outpatient basis or faster than suspected and perhaps of sufficient gravity to merit urgent referral.

There may be anaemia with lymphopenia and leucopenia and the ESR or plasma viscosity may be high. Liver function tests may show non-specific abnormalities. Requests for antibody testing should be accompanied by comprehensive clinical information so that the range of tests performed by the laboratory is appropriate. In cases with predominant arthralgia, where rheumatoid arthritis is a possible diagnosis, rheumatoid factor is clearly of interest, although it may also be positive in almost a fifth of patients with SLE.[3] However, antinuclear antibodies in titres considered significant by the laboratory, supported by a positive profile of additional autoantibodies, will confirm a diagnosis of SLE.[5]

Proteinuria may be quantitated by a 24 hr collection or, more conveniently for the patient, some laboratories may be prepared to measure the protein/creatinine ratio on a random urine sample.[11] Serum electrolyte samples may show high serum creatinine levels indicating significant renal impairment. Even if the serum creatinine is strictly within the normal range at the time of the first blood test, progressive renal failure may still be developing and this will be confirmed by a rising trend in serum creatinine if the blood test is repeated a few days later. Patients with any evidence of renal involvement need urgent specialist referral by telephone. If a diagnosis of SLE has been confirmed by serological methods some centres do not proceed to renal biopsy but others do and may repeat the biopsy after a period of treatment.[12] Fortunately this procedure is relatively atraumatic if fine, mechanically fired biopsy needles are introduced under ultrasound control. Bleeding disorders should be excluded before the procedure and the blood pressure should be as near normal as possible.

Management

Mild forms of SLE

For the mildest forms of SLE which are increasingly recognised, symptomatic treatment may be adequate for some time. Arthralgia may respond to simple analgesics, soluble aspirin or nonsteroidal anti-inflammatory drugs such as diclofenac or naproxen. The photosensitive rash may be minimised by avoiding sunlight but this can be difficult for young women taking an active part in family life. Whilst ultraviolet B of wavelength 280–315 nm is most likely to aggravate a photosensitive skin rash, UVA at wavelength 315–400 nm, even if emitted by fluorescent lights and sunbeds, can also do this. A maximum sunblock cream of Factor 15 or greater is a valuable precaution for the sensitive person, even on overcast days.

The antimalarial drugs, hydroxychloroquine and chloroquine, are helpful in some patients with arthralgia and pleuritic pain and are particularly indicated for rashes with a photosensitive element. They should be discontinued if they cause skin rashes. Their use needs to be monitored with particular caution because of their potential for binding to retinal pigment and causing ocular damage. Eye examination should be performed before starting treatment and this should include visual acuity, central visual field assessment and fundoscopy. If daily doses are kept at or below 400 mg for hydroxychloroquine and 250 mg for chloroquine the chance of visual disturbance is much reduced so that reassessment can be performed perhaps every 6–12 months. If doses need to be increased for any reason, for example to control a flare-up in the disease, eye checks should be performed every 3–4 months. Loss of acuity to red is usually detected earlier than other visual signs after which there may be generalised loss of visual acuity or scotomata because of maculopathy. Corneal opacities may also occur, sometimes causing haloed or blurred vision and these resolve if treatment is stopped. After about 18 months of treatment with antimalarial drugs it is prudent for them to be discontinued for a period of 6 months, even if they have been beneficial in controlling symptoms, to prevent undue drug accumulation.

The clinical expression of SLE is influenced by the sex of the patient but the effect of additional female hormones is unpredictable. It is wise to avoid even low dose oestrogen-containing oral contraceptives but the progestogen-only pills seem safe. Intrauterine devices should be avoided if there is thrombocytopenia.

More severe disease

Corticosteroids underpin the management of more aggressive disease. Typically an initial dose of prednisolone 40–60 mg daily might be used, perhaps even preceded by several doses of intravenous methylprednisolone as an inpatient.[13] Patients on such treatment need a lot of support from family, friends, professional colleagues and their doctors. They need to come to terms as quickly as possible with the loss of good health, adapt their life styles to cope with their symptoms and adjust to the reality of a serious chronic illness which will make them dependent upon medical services for the indefinite future. Many patients will go through philosophical, spiritual and domestic crises at this stage, make their first will and become depressed. In such circumstances patients needs to feel that there is someone who can put these difficulties into perspective and resolve them one by one. This must surely be the GP.

The young woman may be anxious to know whether the disease will have an effect on her ability to have children. She will need to be reassured that she will not pass the disease on to her offspring although, rarely, there may be the risk of congenital heartblock. There is rarely an absolute contra-indication to pregnancy and the outcome is likely to be good for those with mild disease which remits or is controlled by minimal treatment. The outlook is more guarded for aggressive disease requiring several drugs in high dose to control it, if there is severe hypertension, a thrombotic tendency or progressive renal disease.[14] For a young woman the weight gain, altered facial appearance and mood disturbance caused by high dose steroid treatment can also be particularly distressing.

Reducing steroid treatment always poses a dilemma. High initial doses need to be brought down as soon as possible but not if this carries risk of relapse. In practice the dose of prednisolone is reduced progressively over several weeks or months whilst the patient is carefully monitored for recurrence of symptoms. At the same time a spectrum of blood tests is performed at repeated intervals to check that abnormalities previously detected and then suppressed by treatment do not recur.

Patients may continue to experience adverse effects of prednisolone even at doses of less than 20 mg daily, and they often complain of worrying insomnia and agitation. They are usually grateful and relieved when the dose has been reduced over several months to a maintenance level of 5-10 mg daily. They will still need careful supervision and emotional support, they will need to be aware of the possibility of relapse and they will need to know that low dose prednisolone should probably not be stopped without careful consideration, even if they feel very well.

With the slightest new symptom patients may become anxious that their disease has recurred but they may be reluctant to bother their doctor. They need to be reassured that urgent visits to the doctor are part of the process of learning about their own disease and how to manage it, even though some visits will be false alarms. Fever, malaise, fatigue and myalgia might well be part of an intercurrent viral illness but they could equally indicate a flare in disease activity or a more significant bacterial infection resulting from the combined immunosuppressive effects of the disease and its treatment. If infection is a possibility, blood, urine and sputum cultures should be sent to the laboratory direct from the practice and treatment started with broad spectrum antibiotics. Some cases, because of illness and doubt about the diagnosis, will need hospital admission. If the clinical picture is clearly one of early disease relapse it is expedient for the GP to have agreed with his hospital counterpart upon a plan to deal with it. An increase in prednisolone from a maintenance dose of 5–10 mg to a suppressive dose of 20-30 mg might well be satisfactory.

In addition to prednisolone, further treatments may be necessary in some cases of SLE. Patients with more aggressive disease, particularly with nephritis, may need cytotoxic drugs or even plasmapharesis from an early stage. Cyclophosphamide may be more effective in uncontrolled disease than azathioprine but carries the risks of sterility and an increased risk of neoplasia later in life which patients will need to come to terms with. These problems can be minimised if cyclophosphamide is changed to azathioprine as soon as the disease comes under control. Patients on these treatments need very careful supervision and regular blood counts, at weekly intervals initially, which can be arranged by the practice. Cyclophosphamide, azathioprine and the antimalarials also have a steroid sparing effect which may help to minimise the long term complications of high dose prednisolone.

Hypertension must be controlled to minimise renal damage and a combination of antihypertensive drugs may be necessary to keep the blood pressure at an acceptable level. This can be monitored by the GP and his practice nurse, the results being recorded on a co-operation card which is also used in the hospital clinic.

Some symptoms may need additional treatment, either during the early period of disease suppression or in the long term in resistant cases. For example, troublesome Raynaud's phenomenon may improve with slow release nifedipine in doses of 10–60 mg daily. Epilepsy may be controlled with standard anticonvulsant treatments such as phenytoin and carbamazepine. In this respect it is interesting that although an SLE-like syndrome can be induced in susceptible individuals by anticonvulsants and other drugs, the same substances can be used in spontaneous SLE without risk of exacerbating the disease.

Conclusion

Until recently, much of the care for the multisystem rheumatic diseases has been hospital based. Greater confidence in diagnosis and management might be achieved in primary care using a model in which a partner elects to specialise in rheumatology, liaising with the local rheumatologist over complex cases and developing a wider understanding and experience. Principles derived from the management of rheumatoid arthritis are readily transferable to the rarer rheumatic diseases such as SLE. These include support and counselling of the patient and family, monitoring disease activity, adjusting treatments to suppress disease activity and offering specific therapy for symptoms.

References

1. Symmons DPM. Review of UK data on the rheumatic diseases-8: SLE. *Br J Rheumatol* 1991; **30**: 288–90.
2. Dickson DJ. Primary care management of rheumatoid disease. *This volume.*
3. Cervera R, Khamashta MA, Font J, Sebastian GD et al. Systemic lupus erythematosus: clinical and immunologic patterns of disease expression

in a cohort of 1000 patients. *Medicine* 1993; **72**: 113–24.

4. Worrall JG, Snaith ML, Batchelor JR, Isenberg DA. SLE: a rheumato-logical view. Analysis of the clinical features, serology and immuno-genetics of 100 SLE patients during long-term follow-up. *Q J Med* 1990; **74**: 319–30.

5. Charles PJ, Maini RN. Autoantibodies as diagnostic and prognostic indicators in rheumatic and connective tissue diseases. *This volume*, Ch 9

6. Mulherin D, Bresnihan B. Systemic lupus erythematosus. *Baillière's Clin Rheumatol* 1993; **7**: 31–57.

7. Andrews M, Edmunds M, Campbell A, Walls J, Feehally J. Systemic vasculitis in the 1980s – is there an increasing incidence of Wegener's granulomatosis and microscopic polyarteritis? *J R Coll Physicians Lond* 1990; **24**: 284–8.

8. Hunder GG, Arend WP, Bloch DA, Calabrese LH et al. The American College of Rheumatology 1990 criteria for the classification of vasculi-tis. *Arthritis Rheum* 1990; **33**: 1065–7.

9. Conn DL. Update on systemic necrotising vasculitis. *Mayo Clin Proc* 1989; **64**: 535–43.

10. Wong KL, Woo EKW, Wong RWS. Neurological manifestations of systemic lupus erythematosus: a prospective study. *Q J Med* 1991; **81**: 857–70.

11. Ginsberg JM, Chang BS, Matarese RA, Garella S. Use of single voided urine samples to estimate quantitative proteinuria. *N Engl J Med* 1983; **309**: 1543–6.

12. Esdaile JM, Federgreen W, Quintal H, Suissa S, Hayslett JP, Kashgarian M. Predictors of one year outcome in lupus nephritis: the importance of renal biopsy. *Q J Med* 1991; **81**: 907–18.

13. Lockshin MD. Therapy for systemic lupus erythematosus. *N Engl J Med* 1991; **324**: 189–91.

14. Editorial. Systemic lupus erythematosus in pregnancy. *Lancet* 1991; **338**: 87–8.

9 | Autoantibodies as diagnostic and prognostic indicators in rheumatic and connective tissue diseases

PJ Charles and RN Maini
The Kennedy Institute of Rheumatology and the Department of Rheumatology, Charing Cross Hospital, London

Many rheumatic and connective tissue diseases are characterised by one or more autoantibodies directed against cellular antigens. These diseases include systemic lupus erythematosus (SLE), drug-induced lupus erythematosus, Sjögren's syndrome, scleroderma, rheumatoid arthritis (RA), mixed connective tissue disease (MCTD) and dermatomyositis/polymyositis. The autoantibodies may act as specific disease markers, even though the roles of their respective antigens within cells may not be fully understood. Current methodologies for detecting autoantibodies and characterising their antigens have led to a greater knowledge of intracellular processes as well as to a wider range of useful tests for diagnosis, prognosis, and monitoring of disease activity. Some examples of these tests are reviewed here.

Terminology

The terminology for specific autoantibodies and their antigens can be rather confusing. Some autoantibodies are true antinuclear antibodies (ANAs) in that their specific antigen resides within the nucleus, but for others their antigen is located within the cell cytoplasm. Some antigens are named according to their biochemical nature, such as ribonucleoproteins (RNP), single stranded deoxyribonucleic acid (ssDNA) and double stranded DNA (dsDNA). Others have been named according to the diseases in which they occur, such as SS–A in Sjögren's syndrome and PM–1 in polymyositis. Anti-Sm was first described in a patient called 'Smith' suffering from SLE.

Researchers working independently have sometimes given different names to the same antigen. Thus the Mo antigen is the same as nuclear RNP (nRNP) and now called U1-RNP because of its uridine content. Of the Sjögren's syndrome antigens, SS-A is identical to the Ro antigen and SS-B is also known as the La or Ha antigen. The SS-C antigen has been renamed the rheumatoid arthritis-associated nuclear antigen (RANA). The names of some antigens have changed with increasing understanding of their nature. Thus the Scl-1 antigen was renamed Scl-70 because of its molecular weight of 70 kd. The extractable nuclear antigen complex (ENA) was a term applied to antigens which could be extracted in phosphate buffered saline (pH 7.2). ENA was thought to consist of Sm and RNP antigens but many other nuclear and also cytoplasmic antigens are known to be extracted by the same method. The term 'soluble cellular antigens' is a more accurate description.

Sensitivity and specificity

Results of tests need to be accurate, reliable, quality controlled[1] and clinically meaningful. The ideal diagnostic assay, for example, should be highly specific for the disease in question and it should also be highly sensitive by giving a clearly positive result in the great majority of patients with the disorder. Whether this ideal can be achieved depends upon various circumstances. In some situations, as with rheumatoid factor (RF), diagnostic sensitivity may vary with the stage and activity of the disease and the modifying effect of drug treatments. Sensitivity and specificity of a test may also vary with the laboratory technique, so clinicians should be aware of the methods used locally. Thus, enzyme linked immunosorbent assays (ELISA) are more sensitive than those using gel precipitation. Sensitivity may also be affected by genetic background. A notable example occurs in SLE where anti-Sm is twelve times more frequently positive in black compared with white populations.[2] Unfortunately, increased sensitivity often goes hand in hand with decreased specificity, the detection of smaller amounts of antibody possibly leading to mistakenly positive diagnosis in people who do not have the disease.

Specificity of a test is usually assessed against a control population of healthy subjects. Age may also need to be taken into account and, as some autoantibodies occur in healthy elderly people, a suitable age-matched control population should be used. It is sometimes more relevant to evaluate a test in the clinical situation where it is likely to be used. For example, a test group with SLE might be compared to controls with RA where similar clinical features make it part of the differential diagnosis. Technically, the specificity of an assay for detecting antibodies may be affected by materials used as the antigenic source. This may be simply a matter of purity or possibly a more fundamental chemical problem such as the nature and conformation of the peptides present in the assay. The inverse relationship between specificity and sensitivity may also mean that an assay with very high sensitivity may be of little diagnostic use because of its very low specificity.

Antinuclear antibodies

The clinician wishing to assess a patient with a rheumatic or connective tissue disease may be uncertain about current strategies for antibody testing. Full clinical information will allow the laboratory to offer its expertise in the most helpful way. Sera are usually screened initially for ANAs by indirect immunofluorescence (IF) using either cultured human epithelial Hep-2 cells or cryostat sections of rodent tissues. A positive IF-ANA needs to be interpreted with some care. A low titre may occur in about 4% of normal young people but the incidence rises to a fifth in those over 65 years of age. Drugs implicated in the induction of ANAs include not only procainamide and hydralazine but also d-penicillamine, sulphasalazine, chlorpromazine, isoniazid, ethosuximide and phenytoin.

Antigens include ssDNA, dsDNA, deoxyribonucleoprotein (DNP) and histones. Antibodies have also been described against soluble, centromeric and various nucleolar proteins. Such ANAs can be characterised further by the use of techniques such as radio-immunoassay, gel diffusion, ELISA, and immunoblotting. With these methods, ANAs are detectable in nearly all cases of active SLE and MCTD and in about three quarters of cases of Sjögren's syndrome and polymyositis. ANA positivity is unusual in rheumatoid arthritis at the time of presentation but it may occur later in about half the cases, particularly in those with chronic severe joint disease and those with extra-articular involvement.

According to clinical suspicion a particular ANA profile may be tested for. In SLE, sera may be positive for perhaps three or more autoantibodies whereas in scleroderma they are rarely positive for more than one. ANAs which are highly specific to a disease process and rarely found in other circumstances are diagnostically valuable as disease markers (Table 1). They include anti-dsDNA and anti-Sm in SLE and anti-Scl-70 in diffuse scleroderma. Anticentromere antibodies (ACAs) act as useful markers for the limited form of scleroderma, the CRST syndrome with calcinosis, Raynaud's phenomenon, sclerodactyly and telangiectasia. Anti-tRNA synthetases are specific for polymyositis. ANAs are also associated with specific

Table 1. Autoantibodies as disease markers in rheumatic diseases

Antibody Specificity	Disease	Frequency	
dsDNA	SLE	60%	high
Sm	SLE	55% (black) 5% (caucasoid)	high
La(SS-B)	Sjögren's Syndrome	50%	high
SCL-70	Scleroderma	27%	high
Jo-1	Polymyositis	25%	high
Proteinase 3	Wegener's granulomatosis	80%	high
Centromere	CRST syndrome	70%	moderate
nRNP	MCTD	90%	low
Ro(SS-A)	Sjögren's syndrome, SLE	60%	low

clinical features and can help with case management (Table 2). These ANAs are considered in more detail below.

Anti-Ro antibodies

Antibodies to the Ro antigen were first described in primary Sjögren's syndrome, the sicca syndrome not associated with other connective tissue diseases, and occur in 60–80% of cases as well as 1% of normal healthy controls. They are an important finding in SLE, occurring in 40% of patients and tending to be associated with a number of clinical subsets such as the ANA-negative SLE syndrome, subacute cutaneous lupus erythematosus and the lupus-like syndrome associated with homozygous complement C2 and

Table 2. Autoantibodies associated with clinical and pathological features

Antibody	Feature	Comment
dsDNA	diffuse glomerulonephritis	SLE with nephritis
Ro, Sm	membranous glomerulonephritis	SLE with nephritis
Ro	neonatal heart block	maternal antibody
Ro	SLE-vasculitis	
nRNP	Raynaud's phenomenon	as part of overlap syndrome
nRNP, Jo-1	fibrosing alveolitis	overlap, especially Raynaud's
nRNP, Jo-1	polymyositis	with fibrosing alveolitis
La	Sjögren's syndrome	

C4 deficiency. They are also associated with the appearance of nephritis, vasculitis, lymphadenopathy and leukopenia in SLE. In patients negative for dsDNA, levels of anti-Ro antibody serve as an index of disease activity. In SLE cases with anti-Ro who also have anti-DNA antibodies, the renal disease tends to be more aggressive.

Foetal congenital heart block occurs in 5% of all pregnant women who have circulating anti-Ro antibodies and this figure rises to 25% in women with one or more children already affected.[3] This suggests a subgroup of antibodies to Ro directed against cardiac conducting tissue.

Anti-La antibodies

Antibodies to La are found in about half to two thirds of patients with primary Sjögren's syndrome. In the absence of antibodies associated with SLE they are a useful diagnostic marker for primary Sjögren's syndrome where they are found most commonly in patients with extra-glandular features. In SLE, patients with anti-La antibodies tend to have a later age of onset and a lower incidence of nephritis than other cases.[4]

Anti-Sm and nRNP (U1-U6) antibodies

These are antibodies to the protein antigens found in the uridine rich ribonucleuprotein fractions: U1, U2 and U4-6. They include anti-Sm and anti-nRNP, which are often found in combination. The Sm and nRNP antigens are proteins complexed with small nuclear RNAs.

Anti-Sm is found in SLE but prevalence varies with race. In caucasoid populations it is relatively rare with a frequency of only 5% whereas in black populations it rises to 70%.[2] Antibodies to Sm are rarely present in other connective tissue diseases. They therefore serve as a useful marker for SLE, although they do not seem to identify a particular clinical subset.

Anti-nRNP antibodies are found in a variety of connective tissue diseases. They are present in low titres in 10% of patients with SLE, 10% of cases with scleroderma and in some patients with Raynaud's phenomenon and fibrosing lung disease. They also occur in some patients with undifferentiated connective tissue disease and in overlap syndromes in which patients show combined features of two diseases such as SLE and scleroderma, SLE and RA or scleroderma and dermatomyositis.

Anti-nRNP antibodies are particularly useful in the diagnosis of MCTD and were partly responsible for defining it as a specific disease. It is quite different from overlap syndromes although it does incorporate elements of SLE, scleroderma and polymyositis. For these reasons some experts have cast doubt on the validity of the concept of MCTD as a distinct clinical syndrome. Patients tend to have polyarthralgia or arthritis, Raynaud's phenomenon, myositis, oesophageal dysfunction and fusiform swelling of the fingers. High titres of anti-nRNP in the absence of other ANAs are typical of MCTD and are found in 80% of patients.

Anti-ribosomal RNP antibodies

Antibodies to ribosomal RNP (rRNP) or ribosomal P protein are present in approximately 15% of cases of SLE. They were originally described as a marker for neuropsychiatric SLE, but they are more likely to be a marker for active generalised disease.[5]

Anti-double stranded DNA antibodies

Antibodies to dsDNA recognise determinants on the backbone of the DNA helix whereas anti-ssDNA antibodies are directed against the nucleotide bases of the molecule. Anti-dsDNA antibodies are of diagnostic importance in that they are found almost exclusively in SLE, occurring in 60–70% of patients with active disease.[6] Immune complexes of dsDNA and anti-dsDNA may be implicated in the pathogenesis of SLE and particularly in lupus nephritis. They are also extremely important in monitoring disease activity. Increasing antibody levels predict and correlate with increasing disease activity and are often coupled with a decrease in complement C3 and C4 levels, indicating complement consumption.[7] The measurement of antibodies to ssDNA is not helpful as they are nonspecific and are also present in nonrheumatic diseases.

Anti-Scl-70 antibodies

These antibodies, directed against DNA topoisomerase 1, are found in 30% of patients with diffuse scleroderma, a condition with proximal as distinct from localised distal cutaneous disease, with or without systemic manifestations, and synonymous with progressive systemic sclerosis. They are particularly likely in those with more severe skin, joint and lung involvement and are found less frequently in those with more limited scleroderma, such as the CRST syndrome which makes up 20-30% of all cases. They do serve as a useful disease marker because they are not usually present in other connective tissue disorders. Their presence in Raynaud's phenomenon or limited scleroderma may indicate the development of a more severe form of the disease.[8]

Anti-centromere antibodies

ACAs directed against proteins of the centromere complex are found in about 30% of patients with scleroderma. The frequency rises to 80-90% in the subgroup of patients, typically older women, with the CRST syndrome.[9] Occasionally ACAs are found in primary biliary cirrhosis, where half of such cases will also show features of scleroderma.

Anti-nucleolar antibodies

Anti-nucleolar antibodies are a group of antibodies reacting with diverse antigens located within the nucleolar region of the cell including 6-7S RNA, RNA polymerase 1, fibrillarin and U3 RNA. All of these antibodies are present in low frequencies in scleroderma. Another anti-nucleolar antibody, PM-1 or PM/Scl is found in patients with features of polymyositis and scleroderma. Anti-nucleolar antibodies in low titre are occasionally seen in other connective tissue diseases.

Anti-Jo-1 antibodies

Anti-Jo-1 antibodies, directed against histidyl tRNA synthetase, are found in 20% of patients with primary polymyositis, especially the subset with pulmonary fibrosis and arthritis. Interestingly, they do not seem to be a marker for idiopathic pulmonary fibrosis alone. Antibodies have also been described to five other tRNA synthetases: threonyl, alanyl, isoleucyl, glycyl and lysyl. All are associated with a similar clinical syndrome to Jo-1, but are rare, each occurring in less than 4% of polymyositis patients.

Anti-Ku antibodies

Antibodies to the two acidic DNA-binding Ku proteins were originally described in an overlap syndrome with features of polymyositis and scleroderma. They are found in over a third of cases of SLE and scleroderma, in over half with MCTD and also in some patients with Sjören's syndrome and myositis.[10] Further studies are needed to clarify their clinical value.

Antibodies to proliferating cell nuclear antigen

Antibodies to proliferating cell nuclear antigen (cyclin) are a specific marker for SLE, being found in 5% of cases, They are not associated with any particular clinical feature.[11]

ANAs in rheumatoid arthritis

Antibodies to RANA are present in high titres in a majority of patients with RA and in low titres in other rheumatic diseases and normal controls. Their detection, which depends upon the use of cell lines transformed by the Epstein-Barr virus, raises interesting questions about the relationship between this virus and rheumatoid disease. The recently described RA-33 antibodies occur in 30% of patients with RA and 1% of other connective tissue diseases.[12] They may become detectable in RA before other auto-antibodies and may be found in patients who are persistently RF negative.[13]

Rare ANAs

An increasing number of rare spontaneously occurring ANAs are being described in polymyositis, SLE, scleroderma, RA, Sjögren's syndrome and MCTD. Whilst their clinical significance needs to be clarified they also act as useful tools for studying cell function.

Other autoantibodies

Anti-phospholipid antibodies

The anti-phospholipid antibodies (APLAs) include the lupus antico-agulant and anti-cardiolipin antibodies and are responsible for the biological false positive serological test for syphilis. They are common in patients with SLE but may occur without other evidence of collagen, vasculitic or rheumatic diseases. Although the lupus anti-coagulant was first described in SLE complicated by haemorrhage, later work has shown a paradoxical association with thrombosis.

This is a major feature of the anti-phospholipid antibody syndrome which is now recognised as a distinct clinical entity. This syndrome may occur in the absence of features of SLE and such patients may be ANA-negative. Recurrent venous thromboses may lead to pulmonary emboli and pulmonary hypertension whilst repeated arterial thromboses may result in stroke, coronary, peripheral and mesenteric ischaemia. Some cases have thrombocytopaenia, haemolytic anaemia with a positive Coombs test and the lattice-like pattern of dilated superficial veins typical of livido reticularis.[14] Anti-cardiolipin antibodies and lupus anticoagulant may be useful marker for the distressing complication of recurrent foetal loss.[15,16] This tends to occur in the first and second trimesters, possibly resulting from an effect of APLAs on the placenta, but fertility is unimpaired.

Anti-neutrophil cytoplasmic antibodies

Antibodies directed against white cells have long been recognised in RA but for the past ten years they have been found in association with vasculitis involving the small and medium-sized arteries, particularly of the respiratory tract and kidneys. These antineutrophil cytoplasmic antibodies (ANCAs) have now become valuable as disease markers and as indices of disease activity. The ANCA associated with 80% of cases of active Wegener's granulomatosis (WG) localises to the cell cytoplasm on IF and hence is termed C-ANCA. It is directed against proteinase 3, an enzyme in the primary granules which denatures elastin and bacteria as well as having a role in cell differentiation. Rising levels of C-ANCAs are usually associated with an increase in disease activity and persistence of C-ANCA after treatment with prednisolone and cyclophosphamide indicates an increased risk of relapse.[17]

A second antibody pattern, P-ANCA, produces a perinuclear staining pattern on IF and was first associated with necrotising asculitis and rapidly progressive glomerulonephritis. It is found in polyarteritis nodosa, renal vasculitis and the Churg-Strauss syndrome which is characterised by asthma, fever, eosinophilia and necrotising granulomata. It is most frequently directed against myeloperoxidase in primary granules which, on incorporation into lysosomes, oxidises harmful enzymes and destroys bacteria.

Recent work suggests that ANCAs may be implicated in a wider range of disease processes. Antibodies to the lactoferrin enzyme in neutrophil secondary granules may occur in glomerulonephritis and, along with antibodies to myeloperoxidase, may be associated with the vasculitis of RA.[18,19] Other ANCAs await further characterisation.

Rheumatoid factors (RFs)

Of the RFs belonging to the three main classes of immunoglobulin only the IgM RF is measured routinely by most laboratories. It becomes positive in about 80% of cases of RA but it may also be positive in other connective tissue and chronic inflammatory disorders and with increasing age, so a firm diagnosis of RA still depends upon the typical pattern of joint involvement. The level of IgM RF is not a good indicator of disease activity but high titres do tend to occur in aggressive rheumatoid disease with a poor prognosis.

Recent studies looking at other RFs have suggested that levels of IgA RF correlate with cartilage loss, bone erosion, and disease activity.[20] IgG RFs have been associated with vasculitis, but so far they do not have a role in diagnosis and management.[21]

Anti-perinuclear antibodies

Antibodies against the perinuclear granules in human buccal mucosa cells are found in 78% of patients with classical RA and also in 40% of cases with seronegative RA, where they are said to carry a poor prognosis.[22] Clinical use of this assay will not be possible until a satisfactory cultured cell substrate is found to replace human donor cells.

Conclusion

The immunology of connective tissue and rheumatic diseases is a rapidly developing field. Many recent observations have added to its complexity, raising important questions about autoantibodies as causes, markers and monitors of disease. At the same time, characterisation of autoantibodies and their corresponding antigens has given valuable insights into cellular function at a molecular level. Some autoantibodies have helped to define disease entities, some have become established in the process of diagnosis and disease management and others have yet to be explored. For each new autoantibody test which becomes suitable for a specific clinical purpose, the clinician will need to be fully informed and the local laboratory will need a robust and reliable assay.

References

1. Charles PJ, van Venrooij WJ, Maini RN. The consensus workshops for the detection of autoantibodies to intracellular antigens in rheumatic diseases 1989–1992. *Clin Exp Rheum* 1992; **10**: 507–11.
2. Field M, Williams DG, Charles PJ, Maini RN. Specificity of anti-SM antibodies by ELISA for systemic lupus erythematosus: increased sensitivity of detection using purified peptide antigens. *Ann Rheum Dis* 1988; **47**: 820–5.
3. Ramsey–Goldman R, Hom D, Deng J-S. Anti-SS-A antibodies and foetal outcome in maternal systemic lupus erythematosus. *Arthritis Rheum* 1986; **29**: 1269–73.
4. Maddison PJ, Isenberg DA, Goulding NJ, Leddy J, Skinner RP. Anti La (SS-B) identifies a distinct subgroup of systemic lupus erythematosus. *Br J Rheum* 1988; **27**: 27–31.
5. Teh LS, Bedwell AE, Isenberg DA et al. Antibodies to P protein in systemic lupus erythematosus. *Ann Rheum Dis* 1992; **51**: 489–94.
6. Maini RN, Charles PJ, Venables PJW. Antinuclear antibodies in the immunotaxonomy of connective tissue disease. *Scan J Rheumatol* 1984; **56 (suppl)**: 49–57.
7. Swaak AJG, Groenwold J, Bronsveld W. Predictive value of complement profiles and anti-dsDNA in systemic lupus erythematosus. *Ann Rheum Dis* 1986; **45**: 359–66.
8. Kallenberg CGM, Wouda AA, Hoet MH, van Venrooij WJ. Development of connective tissue disease in patients presenting with Raynaud's phenomenon: a six year follow up with emphasis on the predictive value of antinuclear antibodies as detected by immunoblotting. *Ann Rheum Dis* 1988; **44**: 664–71.
9. Steen VD, Powell DL, Medsger TA. Clinical correlations and prognosis based on serum autoantibodies in patients with systemic sclerosis. *Arthritis Rheum* 1988; **31**: 196–203.
10. Yaneva M, Arnett FC. Antibodies against Ku protein in sera from patients with autoimmune disease. *Clin Exp Immunol* 1989; **76**: 255–60.
11. Fritzler MJ, McCarty GA, Ryan JP, Kinsella TD. Clinical features of patients with antibodies directed against proliferating cell nuclear antigen. *Arthritis Rheum* 1983; **26**: 140–5.
12. Hassfield W, Steiner G, Hartmuth K, Smolen JS. Demonstration of a new antinuclear antibody (anti RA33) that is highly specific for rheumatoid arthritis. *Arthritis Rheum* 1989; **32**: 1515–20.
13. Smolen JS, Hassfield W, Graininger W, Steiner G. Antibodies to antinuclear antibody subsets in systemic lupus erythematosus and rheumatoid arthritis. *Clin Exp Rheum* 1990; **8 (Suppl)**: 41–4.
14. Sammaritano LR, Gharavi AE. Antiphospholipid antibody syndrome. *Clin Lab Med* 1992; **12**: 41–55.
15. Love PE, Santaro SA. Antiphospholipid antibodies: anticardiolipin and the lupus anticoagulant in systemic lupus erythematosus (SLE) and in non-SLE disorders. Prevalence and clinical significance. *Ann Intern Med* 1990; **112**: 682–98.
16. Derksen RH, Hasselaar P, Blokzijl L, Gmelig Meyling FH, De Groot PG. Coagulation screen is more specific than the anticardiolipin

ELISA in defining a thrombotic subset of lupus patients. *Ann Rheum Dis* 1988; **47**: 364–71.

17. Hagen EC, Ballieux BEPB, Daha MR, Van Es LA, Van der Woude FJ. Fundamental and clinical aspects of anti-neutrophil cytoplasmic antibodies (ANCA). *Autoimmunity* 1992; **11**: 199–207.

18. Charles PJ, Maini RN. ANCA in rheumatoid arthritis. *Br J Rheum* 1992; **31 (suppl 2)**: 206.

19. Savige JA, Gallicchio MC, Stockman A et al. Anti-neutrophil cytoplasm antibodies in rheumatoid arthritis. *Clin Exp Immunol* 1991; **86**: 92–8.

20. Eberhardt KB, Truedsson L, Pettersson H. Disease activity and joint damage progression in early rheumatoid arthritis: relation to IgG, IgA and IgM rheumatoid factor. *Ann Rheum Dis* 1990; **49**: 906–9.

21. Robbins DL, Feigal DW, Leek JC. Relationship of serum IgG rheumatoid factor to IgM rheumatoid factor and disease activity in rheumatoid arthritis. *J Rheumatol* 1986; **13**: 259–62.

22. Weestgeest AAA, Boerbooms AMTh, Jongmans M. Antiperinuclear factor: indicator of more severe disease in seronegative rheumatoid arthritis. *J Rheumatol* 1987; **14**: 893–7.

10 | Nonsteroidal anti-inflammatory drugs

Adam Young
City Hospital, St Albans

For some rheumatological conditions nonsteroidal anti-inflammatory drugs (NSAIDs) are invaluable. In rheumatoid arthritis they
reduce early morning stiffness, pain, joint swelling and temperature
and thus improve joint function. They may be needed in large doses
to treat tophaceous gout until serum urate can be lowered safely
with allopurinol; in ankylosing spondylitis they are often the main-
stay of treatment and in osteorthritis they play an important role
during specific phases of the disease process. They are also used
frequently for symptom control in a wide range of less well defined
musculoskeletal conditions, 85% of long-term NSAID treatment
being initiated by general practitioners. Indeed, NSAIDs were prescribed on 26 million occasions in the UK in 1989.

The NSAIDs can be classified according to their chemical
structure into two main categories. In the *carboxylic acid group*
are: the *acetic acids* (indomethacin, sulindac, diclofenac, tolmetin,
acemetacin); the *salicylic acids* (aspirin, benorylate, diflunisal, sal-
salate); the *propionic acids* (ibuprofen, flurbiprofen, naproxen,
fenbufen, ketoprofen, tiaprofenic acid, fenoprofen); the *fenamic
acids* (mefanamic acid); the *pyranocarboxylic acids* (etodolac); and the
alkanones (nabumetone). In the *enolic acid group* are: the *benzotri-
azines* (azapropazone); the *oxicams* (piroxicam, tenoxicam) and the
pyrazolones (phenylbutazone).

Surprisingly, the chemical classification of NSAIDs is not very
useful in clinical practice. Despite the apparent similarity of
several NSAIDs, individual variation in response and patient prefer-
ence play a major part in the choice of such drugs in the long term.
Time and patience are often required to tailor the drug and dose
schedule to the needs of the individual.

Adverse effects of NSAIDs

The risks of NSAIDs are such that in the USA they have been
declared a major health care problem and carry a health warning.

There is still controversy over the size of the problem[1] but the cost of investigating and treating complications is said to be enormous. The prevalence of some side effects is shown in Table 1.[2]

Table 1. Prevalence of side effects with common NSAIDs[2]

NSAID	GI	Toxicity (%) CNS	Mucocutaneous
Azapropazone	15.6	8.3	9.4
Benorylate	19.2	8.5	3.7
Diclofenac	17.3	11.7	2.2
Fenbufen	12.7	8.2	10.9
Ibuprofen	14.4	6.0	3.3
Indomethacin	15.2	30.0	1.3
Ketoprofen	24.1	8.9	2.5
Naproxen	12.1	6.9	1.9
Piroxicam	12.4	6.7	2.9
Tiaprofenic acid	15.2	8.9	2.6

Gastrointestinal problems

NSAIDs may cause diarrhoea and also haemorrhage or perforation of the small bowel and colon, but their most notable adverse effects are seen in the stomach and duodenum. Their use is associated with an increased incidence of gastric ulceration and a higher risk of complications from gastric ulceration such as perforation, haemorrhage and death. By contrast, the incidence of duodenal ulceration does not seem to be increased but there is a greater risk of complications if duodenal damage is already present. The individual risk is not high but the widespread use of NSAIDs makes gastroduodenal damage a major problem in the population as a whole and more so in certain patient subgroups. The risk of presenting with upper gastrointestinal bleeding or perforation is about 1.5 times greater than in non-NSAID users.[3]

The mechanisms that lead to NSAID-induced mucosal damage are not completely understood. Endogenous prostaglandins play an important role in mucosal protection by stimulating the secretion of mucus and bicarbonate, maintaining blood flow and binding directly to parietal cells to inhibit acid secretion. NSAIDs exert their adverse effects principally by inhibiting prostaglandin production but some may also have a direct irritant action.[4] Gastroduodenal ulceration may also be commoner in NSAID users positive for *Helicobacter pylori*[3] but the value of specifically treating this has not been studied.

Symptomatic assessment of gastroduodenal complications can be misleading in patients taking NSAIDs. Of those patients with dyspepsia about a fifth have a normal mucosa endoscopically[5] whilst more than 50% of lesions show 'silent mucosal injury'[6] with no symptoms. Endoscopically, mucosal lesions in patients taking NSAIDS might be conveniently categorised as mucosal haemorrhages, erosions and ulcers. The significance of small discrete gastric mucosal haemorrhages is unknown but erosions, where there is a break in the mucosal lining, may progress in size and depth to form ulcers with the attendant risks of haemorrhage and perforation. Even so, with continued administration of NSAIDs, a process of adaptation occurs in many patients so that gastroduodenal mucosal injury lessens with time and may even resolve. This dynamic process of damage with the capacity to heal may partly explain why there is no consistent relationship between the duration of NSAID intake and the occurrence of complications.

Several approaches have been employed to prevent or reduce the gastroduodenal damage resulting from the use of NSAIDs. Histamine H2 receptor antagonists reduce gastric microbleeding induced by aspirin but, contrary to expectation, seem ineffective in preventing gastric mucosal erosions from other NSAIDs. They do appear to reduce the damage from NSAIDs to the duodenal mucosa, although quantitatively this is of less importance than damage to gastric mucosa.[7,8] Omeprazole, a proton pump inhibitor, is effective in healing peptic ulcers resistant to H2 antagonists but it has not been evaluated sufficiently in the context of NSAID-associated damage.

Misoprostol, a synthetic analogue of Prostaglandin E1, does prevent gastric ulceration in patients on NSAIDs,[9] presumably through its cytoprotective effects rather than via the suppression of gastric acid production. A dose of 200 µg twice daily is more effective than 100 µg four times daily. It is also as effective as a dose of 200 µg four times daily but avoids the side effects of abdominal pain, diarrhoea and dyspepsia which might otherwise occur in almost a third of cases.[10] Clinical studies where misoprostol has been coadministered with NSAIDs have shown no reduction in efficacy of the NSAIDs.

Comparative trials indicate that histamine H2 receptor antagonists, sucralfate and misoprostol provide similar protection against duodenal damage whilst misoprostol is better than other treatments in preventing NSAID-induced gastric injury.[11]

In the absence of sufficient long term studies to define good practice, routine prophylaxis against severe symptomatic gastrointestinal damage is unwarranted and unduly costly. However, such treatment

might be prudent in high risk groups such as those who have previously stopped NSAIDs because of gastrointestinal side effects,
patients over 70 years old, those with a history of peptic ulcer within
the previous five years, debilitating conditions such as severe cardiac, renal or hepatic failure, current steroid therapy or those who
smoke.[12]

Renal toxicity

Prostaglandins are involved in various aspects of renal function
including control of blood flow, glomerular filtration, ion transport
and renin release. It is therefore not surprising that NSAIDs should
affect renal function by blocking the actions of prostaglandins as well
as having other direct drug effects. They have been implicated in
acute renal failure, papillary necrosis, acute and chronic inter-stitial
nephritis, the nephrotic syndrome and analgesic nephropathy.[13,14]

NSAIDs have little effect on renal function in normal subjects,
apart from causing a detectable degree of sodium retention. Their
effects become more overt in disease states where high levels of
renin and angiotensin tend to cause vasoconstriction within the
kidney. This tendency is normally opposed by a compensatory
vasodilator effect of prostaglandins. If their beneficial action is
blocked by NSAIDs, renal function may deteriorate quite quickly,
even to the point of acute renal failure which may then be irre-
versible. NSAIDs therefore need to be avoided or used with care in
all renal diseases, especially those with any degree of renal impairment, in cardiac failure, in cirrhosis with ascites, in all conditions
associated with sodium depletion and in the elderly who have
diminished renal reserve. Rheumatic conditions, such as rheumatoid arthritis, systemic lupus erythematosus and scleroderma, may
present dilemmas in management where NSAIDs may need to be
used against a background of progressive renal involvement caused
by the diseases themselves or by the development of amyloid.

In general clinical practice, and if NSAIDs are avoided in the high-
est risk cases, perhaps 10–25% of patients on NSAIDs will develop
oedema,[13] some will show an asymptomatic increase in serum creatinine which is usually reversible[15] and the occasional patient will
become hyperkalaemic because of inhibition of potassium excretion.
It is just as well to check the electrolytes before starting NSAIDs in
any patient potentially at high risk of adverse effects and this would
include the elderly. In such cases, renal function should be monitored by rechecking electrolytes a week or so after starting treatment,
again after 2–3 months and then perhaps twice yearly.

Other adverse effects

Neurological side effects of NSAIDs are quite common and include headache, particularly with indomethacin, dizziness, drowsiness, tinnitus, confusion and euphoria. They may be obtrusive enough to impair concentration and prevent driving. Fortunately these effects are rapidly reversible when treatment is stopped. Mucocutaneous side effects of NSAIDs include an irritating macular skin rash which appears typically after 1–2 weeks of treatment and fades quickly when the drug is stopped. Stomatitis, photosensitivity, urticaria and Stevens-Johnson syndrome occur occasionally. Anaphylaxis, asthma and pulmonary oedema have been described.

A normochromic normocytic anaemia, more or less proportional to the activity of an underlying rheumatic condition, is typical of the anaemia of chronic disease. A hypochromic, microcytic picture in the patient on NSAIDs raises the possibility of iron deficiency anaemia secondary to chronic blood loss from the gastrointestinal tract. Measurement of serum ferritin or bone marrow aspiration may be needed to clarify the situation. Haemolytic anaemia and thrombocytopaenia are rare, as is aplastic anaemia now that phenylbutazone can only be prescribed by rheumatologists for ankylosing spondylitis.

NSAIDs sometimes cause a reversible rise in hepatic transaminases or more rarely hepatocellular damage or cholestatic jaundice. Whether or not they have an adverse effect on cartilage causing aseptic necrosis is still a matter for debate.[1]

Safe prescribing

The wide range of potentially serious drug interactions listed in the appendix of the British National Formulary would seem to make NSAIDs some of the most difficult drugs to use safely. However, some interactions only apply to a small number of drugs in this category and, because of careful vigilance and avoidance of such drugs in high risk groups, the frequency of clinically significant drug interactions is relatively low.[16]

Diuretics may be rendered less effective by NSAIDs, they may enhance the potential nephrotoxicity of NSAIDs and, in the case of potassium conserving diuretics, there may be particular risk of hyperkalaemia. Similarly, there may be increased risk of renal failure and serious hyperkalaemia with ACE inhibitors whilst other antihypertensive drugs may be rendered less effective. Some NSAIDs block the excretion of methotrexate and lithium, thus increasing the possibility of toxicity whilst probenecid has the converse effect of delaying the excretion of some NSAIDs. Effects of sulphonylureas and phenytoin are enhanced by azapropazone and phenylbutazone. Caution is always required when NSAIDs are used at the same time as warfarin, the inhibition of metabolism giving the chance of life-threatening bleeding.

A number of alternative approaches can be used to reduce the dose or even the need for NSAIDs. Patients with inflammatory arthropathies who respond poorly to anti-inflammatory drugs should be considered for second-line drugs sooner rather than later. Physical treatments are often beneficial, such as physiotherapy, manipulation, splintage, transcutaneous nerve stimulation and acupuncture. Pain should also be more easily controllable after explanation and reassurance. Sleep patterns and mood may be improved by a combination of antidepressant and simple analgesic treatment at night. Even so, NSAIDs are of such value in the inflammatory arthropathies that they should not be avoided if the benefits are greatly in excess of the risks.

Conclusion

NSAIDs have an established place in the treatment of inflammatory arthropathies and a variety of other conditions where there is an inflammatory element. Their benefits are offset by a range of adverse effects, particularly an increased chance of gastric ulceration and an increase in complications arising from both gastric and duodenal ulceration. The action of NSAIDs on the kidney may result in a spectrum of renal impairment or altered drug metabolism sufficient to lead to toxicity. Whilst these problem have not been exactly quantitated in size, the widespread and inappropriate use of NSAIDs would suggest that their potential for adverse effects is much greater than it need be. The ratio of benefits to risks could be greatly improved by simple guidelines confining the use of NSAIDs to the conditions for which they are really indicated, by using them for the shortest possible time in individual cases and by avoiding them completely in high risk groups.

References

1. Henry DA. Side-effects of non-steroidal anti-inflammatory drugs. *Baillière's Clin Rheumatol* 1988; **2**: 425–54.
2. Cox NL, Doherty SM. Non-steroidal anti-inflammatories: outpatient audit of patient preferences and side-effects in different diseases.

In: Rainsford KD, Velo GP, eds. *Side effects of anti-inflammatory drugs. 1, Clinical and epidemiological aspects.* Lancaster: MTP Press, 1987: 137–50.

3. Ballinger A. Prevention of peptic ulceration in patients receiving NSAIDs. *B J Hosp Med* 1993; **49**: 767–72.
4. Semble EL, Wu WC. Prostaglandins in the gut and their relationship to non-steroidal anti-inflammatory drugs. *Baillière's Clin Rheumatol* 1989: **3**: 247–69.
5. Scander MP, Ryan FP. Non-steroidal anti-inflammatory drugs and pain free peptic ulcers in the elderly. *Br Med J* 1988; **297**: 833–4.
6. Larkai EN, Smith JL, Lidsky MD, Graham DY. Gastro-duodenal mucosa and dyspeptic sumptoms in arthritic patients during chronic non-steroidal anti-inflammatory drug use. *Am J Gastroenterol* 1987; **82**: 1153–8.
7. Ehsanullah RSB, Page MC, Tildesley G, Wood JR. Prevention of gastro-duodenal damage induced by non-steroidal anti-inflammatory drugs: controlled trial of ranitidine. *Br Med J* 1988; **297**: 1017–21.
8. Robinson M, Mills RJ, Eular AR. Ranitidine prevents duodenal ulcers associated with non-steroidal anti-inflammatory drug therapy. *Aliment Pharmacol Ther* 1991; **5**: 143–50.
9. Graham DY, Agrawal N, Roth SH. Prevention of NSAID-induced gastric ulcer with misoprostol: multicentre double-blind placebo-controlled trial. *Lancet* 1988; **ii**: 1277–80.
10. Lanza FL, Kochman RL, Geis GS, Rack EMF, Deysach LG. A double-blind placebo-controlled 6-day evaluation of two doses of misoprostol in gastroduodenal mucosal protection against damage from aspirin and effect on bowel habits. *Am J Gastroenterol* 1991; **86**: 1743–8.
11. Henry DA. Gastrointestinal bleeding and non-steroidal anti-inflammatory drugs. In: Lawson DH ed. *Current Medicine 3, Royal College of Physicians of Edinburgh.* Edinburgh: Churchill Livingstone, 1991: 171–89.
12. Fries JF, Miller SR, Spitz PW, Williams CA, Hubert HB, Bloch DA. Towards an epidemiology of gastropathy associated with non-steroidal anti-inflammatory drug use. *Gastroenterology* 1989; **96**: 647–55.
13. Clive DM, Stoff JS. Renal syndromes associated with non-steroidal anti-inflammatory drugs. *N Engl J Med* 1984; **310**: 563–72.
14. Adams DH, Morrie AJ, Michael J, McConkey B, Bacon PA, Adu D. Non-steroidal anti-inflammatory drugs and renal failure. *Lancet* 1986; **i**: 57–9.
15. Bird HA. The kidney in rheumatic diseases. *Ann Rheum Dis* 1989; **48**: 1029–30.
16. Buchan IE, Bird HE. Drug interactions in arthritic patients. *Ann Rheum Dis* 1991; **50**: 680–1.

11 | Injection of joints and periarticular tissues

Anthony K Clarke
Royal National Hospital for Rheumatic Diseases, Bath

The steroid injection is a powerful therapeutic tool, highly effective in the use of medical time, easily performed in surgery or clinic and much appreciated by patients. Joints should be considered for injection if affected by sterile inflammatory synovitis, especially if an effusion is also present. Conditions leading to this include rheumatoid arthritis, reactive, psoriatic, colitic and other types of seronegative arthritis, gout and pyrophosphate arthritis. After a single injection, intra-articular steroids are rapidly taken up by synovial cells and clinical improvement may be maintained for weeks or months. Sometimes, pain and swelling are reduced for a much longer period and synovitis may never recur, particularly in small joints of the fingers and toes.

Soft tissue inflammatory lesions are common causes of symptoms. They may result from repeated use, minor trauma, as part of generalised inflammation in rheumatoid disease orsecondary to abnormal joint function in osteoarthritis. They include juxta-articular lesions such as bursitis, capsulitis and ligamentous strain and they respond readily and sometimes permanently to steroid injection, especially if given early. Extra-articular lesions also respond well: entrapment neuropathies, tendinitis, rotator cuff disorders of the shoulder and lesions of bone-tendon junctions. These latter enthesopathies, such as tennis elbow, can be very troublesome; accurate point-tenderness injection will relieve pain and improve mobility greatly in most cases.

Basic technique

Before injection treatment is considered, the diagnosis should be reviewed carefully to exclude referred pain and neuropathic lesions. Joint and periarticular injections are relatively easy to perform, the techniques being learnt best by watching an expert then practising under supervision. An aseptic no-touch technique is essential, using sterile disposable equipment and single-dose ampoules which also reduce the risk of sepsis. Correct siting of the injection requires a knowledge of the local anatomy so access to suitable monographs may be useful if exact details need to be checked.[1,2,3] It is often helpful to mark the injection spot which, in soft tissue lesions, is often at the point of maximum tenderness. If necessary, ethyl chloride can be used for skin analgesia. The injection site should be well swabbed with isopropyl alcohol, iodine or a similar antiseptic and care should be taken not to support the needle with the fingers. The feeling of resistance to injecting the contents of the syringe is a useful guide to correct placement of the needle, especially with soft tissue lesions. With few exceptions, such as tennis elbow, resistance to injection should be low. If it is unexpectedly high, the needle may be in tendon, ligament or periosteum. An injection misplaced in this way can occasionally lead to problems, for example softening and rupture of the long head of the biceps. Partial withdrawal of the needle within the same puncture site and re-exploration at different angles usually results in a satisfactory position. Correct location may be confirmed if an injection containing local anaesthetic rapidly relieves symptoms. For a lesion such as bursitis, aspiration of fluid confirms correct positioning. Fluid should also be aspirated, if possible, before a joint is injected and this should be cultured and examined under the polarizing light microscope for the presence of crystals, as in gout or pyrophosphate arthropathy. Aspiration also relieves pain by reducing pressure within the joint. If infection is suspected the joint should not be injected.

Hydrocortisone acetate was first used for intra-articular and soft-tissue injection, then side-chain modification of the steroid nucleus led to more potent and longer acting analogues. Suitable preparations now include: hydrocortisone acetate (HA) 25 mg/ml; methyl prednisolone acetate (MPA) 40 mg/ml and triamcinolone hexacetonide (THA) 20 mg/ml. They are all micro-crystalline suspensions and rarely they produce a transient gout-like post-injection flare when injected into joints. This crystal-induced inflammation comes on quickly but resolves over 24-48 hours, assisted if necessary by rest and a nonsteroidal anti-inflammmatory drug such as oral indomethacin. The different properties of these steroid preparations can be exploited to advantage in different clinical situations. HA is relatively short-acting whilst MPA and THA are longer acting. MPA and HA are suitable for injection into both superficial and deep sites whereas THA, the most powerful injectable steroid available, should be reserved mostly for deep structures. Superficial injection of THA, especially if repeated and if there is leakage along the needle track, may cause depigmentation of skin and atrophy of both skin and sub-cutaneous tissues.

It is now common practice to inject a steroid and a local anaes-thetic together, the volume of injection being determined very much by the anatomy. In a big joint like the knee, a mixture con-taining a large volume of 9-10 ml of lignocaine 1% will help to distribute the steroid. Much smaller volumes with lower doses of steroid will suit small joints and soft tissues. MPA 40 mg/ml is con-veniently available as a mixture with lignocaine 10 mg/ml (MPAL) and this combination is quite useful where very small volumes are needed. If local anaesthetic is not included in the steroid prepara-tion, lignocaine 1% may be added.

When local anaesthetic is injected with steroid its analgesic effect may wear off quite quickly so patients may be surprised to find that pain gets worse before it gets better. This possibility should be explained before the injection to avoid misunderstanding. After a delay of perhaps 24–48 hours the benefit of the steroid injection then becomes apparent and may continue to increase over 2–3 weeks. Systemic absorption of steroid over this time may improve inflammatory symptoms elsewhere but it may also cause facial flush-ing and worsen glycaemic control in diabetics. If severe pain persists despite a successful injection, infection should be suspected and an attempt made to aspirate the joint or soft tissue. However, if a scrupulous no-touch technique is used infection is more of a theoretical risk.

As a general rule, any one site should not be injected more than three times per year. More frequent injections carry the disad-vantages of adrenal suppression, marked local tissue atrophy and degeneration of underlying cartilage and bone. Aseptic necrosis, which occurs in weight-bearing joints affected by erosive arthritis, is even more likely after frequent steroid injections. For soft tissue lesions, satisfactory but temporary relief might encourage further injections but failure to respond after two injections would suggest a need for alternative treatment. After all, injection therapy is only one aspect of rheumatology care. Repetitive strain lesions which respond well but recur after injection should be reassessed for pre-disposing factors.

Injecting joints and soft tissues

The shoulder

Capsulitis of the shoulder is common and disabling. In the majority, the range of movement is only restricted by pain but in more severe cases there is true limitation of movement: the *frozen shoulder*. This is caused by stiffening of the soft tissues around the joint, leading to what is rather inaccurately called *adhesive capsulitis*. Night pain is frequent and usually means that physiotherapy will be ineffective. Although the problem is essentially periarticular, treatment is by intra-articular injection using HA 25–50 mg or THA 10–20 mg made up to 5 ml with lignocaine 1%. The steroid becomes widely spread throughout the joint and then diffuses into the adjacent soft tissues over the following week or so. In refractory cases this injection can be repeated twice at three weekly intervals.

In a *rotator cuff lesion*, pain and tenderness are localised to the the common insertion of the supraspinatus, infraspinatus, subcapsularis and teres minor muscles. Shoulder movements may be well preserved initially but marked stiffness may develop with time. This may improve with physiotherapy after steroid injection. The rotator cuff is injected via a lateral approach, the needle being directed medially from a point between the tip of the acromion and the head of the humerus. As with capsulitis, HA 25–50 mg or THA 10–20 mg made up to 5 ml with lignocaine 1% is suitable.

In *subacromial bursitis* there is often diffuse swelling of the shoulder and a painful arc syndrome where pain is felt between about 45° and 135° when the arm is brought down laterally from the vertical position. The bursa is easily aspirated and injected using a lateral or anterior approach. The underside of the acromion process is identified and the skin marked about 5 mm below. A 21 gauge (G) 0.8 x 40 mm needle inserted at about 30° from the horizontal will enter the sub-acromial space and HA 25 mg or THA 10–20 mg made up to 5 ml with lignocaine 1% can be injected without resistance.

Rheumatoid arthritis may involve both joints of the shoulder but the *acromioclavicular joint* is more likely to be tender as a result of trauma. It can be injected directly from above and will accommodate a small amount of fluid. THA 2 mg made up to 0.5 ml with lignocaine 1% should be injected through a 19G 1.1 x 50 mm needle.

The *glenohumeral joint*, the true shoulder joint, communicates with the tendon sheath of the long head of the biceps and often with the subacromial bursa. External rotation becomes limited and referred pain may be felt more in the upper arm than the shoulder, extending in more severe cases to the hand and neck. The joint is easily injected using an anterior approach. The joint line is identified with the patient sitting against a back rest. HA 25–50mg or THA 20 mg made up to 5 ml with 1% lignocaine is slowly and gently injected using a 21G 0.8 x 40 mm needle. If there is resistance to injection the needle may be in the long head of the biceps and should be repositioned to avoid rupture of the tendon. The joint may also be injected from behind, the needle being directed from a point below the acromion towards the coracoid process.

The elbow

Enthesopathies at the elbow are common and troublesome. Most cases arise from direct or indirect trauma but some may be soft tissue manifestations of rheumatoid arthritis or a spondyloarthropathy. Steroid injections help most cases of both tennis and golfer's elbow but to be successful the injections needs to be placed accurately into the lesions. Transient post-injection pain may be quite severe so patients should be made aware of this before agreeing to the procedure. For *tennis elbow* the lateral epicondyle and common extensor origin are palpated to find the site of maximum tenderness. To do this, the thumb of the non-operative hand is advanced in a proximal to distal direction. When the most tender area is found, the needle is inserted through clean skin distal to the exploring thumb at an angle of 45° so that the tip lies beneath the thumb. HA 25 mg or MPA 40 mg in 1 ml of lignocaine 1% is injected into the tender area. For *golfer's elbow* the same procedure is applied to the medial epicondyle and common flexor origin.

Olecranon bursitis is painful and aspiration of the bursa plus injection of steroid is usually helpful. *Rheumatoid nodules* at the elbow may also improve dramatically if injected directly with HA 25 mg or MPA 20–40 mg in a small volume of lignocaine 1%.[4]

The *elbow joint*, actually consisting of three joints in communication, the humero-ulnar, radiohumeral and superior radio-ulnar joints, can respond well to intra-articular steroids. With the elbow resting on a table and flexed to 90° the joint space can be penetrated easily using a lateral approach. The radiohumeral joint line is located by feeling the head of the radius whilst rotating the forearm. The needle is then inserted about 1 cm above the lateral epicondyle and the joint injected with HA 25 mg or THA 10–20 mg diluted in 5 ml lignocaine 1%. Alternatively, a posterolateral approach can be used with the elbow flexed to 70°. The depression between the olecranon and the lateral epicondyle is located and the needle directed in a forward and slightly downward plane.

The wrist and hand

Mild degrees of *carpal tunnel syndrome* often respond temporarily or even permanently to steroid injection. A 23G 0.6 x 25 mm needle is inserted superficially in the midline above the distal wrist crease, directed slightly downwards and advanced distally into the palm to a depth of some 5–9 mm. The needle should be withdrawn slightly if symptoms suggest that the median nerve has been touched. HA 25 mg or MPA 40 mg is injected the length of the carpal tunnel as the needle is slowly withdrawn. Local anaesthetic is best avoided as it may cause transient numbness and paralysis. Median nerve symptoms may worsen briefly after injection because of the increased fluid volume in the carpal tunnel but this soon resolves.

Pain arising along the radial border of the wrist is often caused by *de Quervain's stenosing tenovaginitis* involving the common tendon sheath of the extensor pollicis brevis and the abductor pollicis longus. An injection of HA 25 mg or MPA 40 mg in a small volume of perhaps 0.5–1 ml of lignocaine 1% is given into the tendon sheath. It should be possible to see the mixture inflate the tendon sheath as the injection proceeds.

At the wrist, the radio-carpal and inferior radio-ulnar joints are affected by rheumatoid disease and less commonly by osteoarthritis, sometimes secondary to previous trauma. If wrist pain persists despite splinting and rest, it is worth trying an injection into the *radio-carpal joint* using HA 25 mg or THA 10-20 mg made up to 5 ml with lignocaine 1%. Using a dorsal approach the needle is inserted between the lunate and scaphoid bones and advanced towards the end of the radius at an angle of 60° to the skin. The *inferior radio-ulnar joint* often communicates with the radio-carpal joint but it can also be injected separately if necessary. A 23G needle is inserted just beyond the tip of the ulnar styloid and advanced into the joint which is then injected with HA 25 mg or THA 10–20 mg made up to 2 ml with lignocaine 1%.

The *first carpo-metacarpal joint* at the base of the thumb is frequently involved in primary nodal osteoarthritis and responds quite well to injection. A convenient route is through the palmar surface at the base of the thenar eminence, although anterolateral and dorsal routes can also be used. The injection of choice is MPAL 1 ml. The joint space is usually much reduced in osteoarthritis so any benefit may derive from some extra-articular effect of the steroid. Transient post-injection pain may be quite severe.

Tenosiniovitis in the wrist and hand may be associated with rheumatoid arthritis or repeated trauma. The common flexor tendon

sheath of the middle three fingers is usually separate from those of
the thumb and little finger. When inflamed it may be palpable or
visible as a swelling in the palm. THA made up to 2 ml with lignocaine 1% can give relief if injected into the tendon sheath.

In the fingers, *metacarpophalangeal (MCP) and proximal interphalangeal (PIP) joints* affected by rheumatoid arthritis may be injected
with a small amount of steroid, perhaps 0.5-1 ml MPAL, using a 23G
needle. A dorsal or dorsolateral approach is often satisfactory with
the patient seated, hands resting on a table. A palmar approach is
also very easy. Similarly it is also possible to inject *distal interphalangeal (DIP) joints* affected by osteo- or psoriatic arthritis. Injections
into small finger joints can be very painful so ethyl chloride can be
used and only a few joints should be injected at any one sitting.
Painful *Heberden's nodes*, on the terminal phalanges adjacent to
the DIP joints, can be injected individually with 0.5 ml MPAL.
Transient anaesthesia may occur distally if lignocaine affects the
digital nerve.

The back

Fibromyalgia is common and many patients have trigger spots which
are spontaneously painful and exquisitely tender to palpation. Such
areas are often found overlying the lower cervical spine, the medial
borders of the scapulae, the lower lumbar spine and the posterior
iliac crests. A combined treatment programme should aim to
improve sleep and general fitness and might also include tricyclic
antidepressants, physiotherapy and exercises. In addition, the worst
of the trigger spots can be injected with 20 mg THA in 2–3 ml
lignocaine to produce temporary relief.

The hip

Local steroids are rarely indicated for disorders of the hip joint and
the injection is difficult enough to need specialised day surgery
facilities. Soft tissue injections, on the other hand, are an 'office
procedure'. The hip symptoms described by many patients are
frequently localised to the outer aspect of the upper thigh and are
caused by *trochanteric bursitis*. Pain and tenderness are related to the
inflamed bursa overlying the greater trochanter some 10 cm below
the level of the anterior superior iliac spine. The patient should lie
facing the doctor with the painful side uppermost, the hip slightly
flexed and adducted so that the knee rests on the couch in front of
the other leg. The area of maximal tenderness should be marked on

the skin. THA 20 mg or HA 50 mg made up to 10 ml with lignocaine 1% should be injected deeply via a lateral approach into the area of maximal tenderness, using a 21G 0.8 x 40 mm needle.

The ischial tuberosities bear the weight of the body in the sitting position and the overlying bursae and muscle insertions may sometimes become tender. The point of maximum tenderness should be defined, deep in the medial side of the buttocks, with the patient lying face down. *Ischial bursitis* should respond well to THA 10 mg or HA 50 mg made up to 10 ml with lignocaine 1%. Additional benefit may be obtained by infiltrating the surrounding muscle attachments.

The knee

In the knee, ligamentous strain is often secondary to underlying osteoarthritis, even at an early stage. Typically this occurs in ageing women with valgus deformity, lateral instability and persistent pain in the knee on weight bearing. In such cases *medial ligament strain* produces local tenderness at its inferior attachment over the medial aspect of the upper tibia. Local injection of steroid and lignocaine at these points will often relieve pain. Areas of maximal tenderness are identified, marked and injected with 1 ml MPAL. Post-injection pain may last for up to 24 hours. Benefit may be sustained by vigorous quadriceps exercises using weights but may be short-lived if exercise is not maintained and if previous risk factors still prevail, such as obesity and knee deformity.

Inflammatory arthritis and synovitis of the *knee joint* are easily treated, except occasionally in the very obese where large fat pads make entry into the joint cavity more difficult. The knee joint is entered on the medial or lateral side between the patella and femur with the knee joint extended. With the medial approach, for example, the needle is inserted at an angle of 45° towards the centre of the joint about 0.5 cm below the patella. As the needle advances slowly it can be felt to enter the joint cavity. If there is fixed flexion deformity, as in established rheumatoid arthritis, injection is often easier antero-medially below the patella, just beside the patellar tendon with the knee flexed to 90°. To make the knee more comfortable, any effusion should be drained completely, so the needle should be mounted initially on an empty sterile syringe. The synovial fluid should be examined for bacteria and crystals. If there is no suspicion of infection the joint can be injected with HA 100 mg or THA 20 mg made up to 10 ml with lignocaine 1% using a 21G 0.8 x 40 mm needle. This may produce benefit for up to two months but often no longer because of clearance of steroid into the systemic circulation. *Baker's cyst* (the popliteal bursitis described by William Baker in 1877) may be secondary to arthritis at the knee, and as the two structures are in continuity it benefits indirectly from any treatment instilled into the joint. *Prepatellar bursitis*, or housemaid's knee, often responds to an injection into the bursa anterior to the patellar ligament.

The ankle and foot

The *ankle joint* may need injection if inflamed by rheumatoid disease, the seronegative arthropathies or ankylosing spondylitis. It is fairly easy to inject if the foot is plantar flexed as much as possible. The joint line is identified and a 21G 0.8 x 40 mm needle inserted anteriorly, below the distal end of the tibia and just lateral to the tibialis anterior tendon. HA 100 mg or THA 20 mg should be made up to 2-3 ml with lignocaine 1%, but a larger volume of up to 10 ml may help to distribute the steroid in a very swollen joint.

In addition to the ankle joint, other structures around the ankle can become inflamed. Thus, the painful ankle in rheumatoid arthritis is often due to *tenosinovitis of the medial and lateral tendons*. These include the peroneal tendons behind the lateral malleolus, the long extensor tendons in front of the ankle and the tibialis posterior tendon behind the medial malleolus. Swollen tendon sheaths can usually be injected by entering them tangentially beside the tendon using a 21G 0.8 x 40 mm needle mounted on a 2 ml syringe. A mixture of HA 25 mg added to 0.5 ml lignocaine 1%, or MPAL 1 ml, is usually satisfactory.

The Achilles tendon is covered by a thin paratenon rather than a tendon sheath. *Achilles tendinitis* occurs as a result of repeated strain but the tendon and its insertion may be affected by the HLA-B27 associated disorders, ankylosing spondylitis and Reiter's disease as well as gout. Steroid injection is not used here because of the risk of subsequent tendon rupture. By contrast, *Achilles bursitis*, caused by these same conditions and also by rheumatoid arthritis, can be treated by steroid injection. There is a point of maximum tenderness on the posterior aspect of the heel where the bursa lies between the Achilles tendon and the upper border of the calcaneum. The needle passes easily into the bursa and aspiration of highly viscous fluid may be possible. HA 25 mg or THA 10 mg made up to 2 ml with ligniocaine 1% can be injected with prolonged benefit. As usual, aspirated fluid should be sent for analysis.

Pain in the heel, an affliction of long distance runners and policemen, is often due to *plantar fasciitis*. When bilateral it may be associated with Reiter's disease, psoriatic arthropathy and ankylosing spondylitis. It may responds to steroid injection but the outcome is rather unpredictable. Injecting through the sole is difficult and painful so the best approach is laterally or medially through the softer skin, advancing the needle into the foot to the area of maximum tenderness. One or two injections of a mixture containing steroid and lignocaine are given into the point of maximum tenderness, usually medially at the origin of the plantar fascia. This is an uncomfortable injection which the patient should understand in advance. After the injection, the patient should use a sorbo-rubber shoe insert with a hole cut out at the point of maximal tenderness to relieve pressure under the heel.

The *subtalar joint* is best injected from the lateral aspect at a level just above the tip of the lateral malleolus, the needle pointing towards the first metatarsal head. However, if the joint is everted by the valgus deformity of rheumatoid disease, the injection may be difficult. Other *joints of the mid-foot* can be painfully affected by osteoarthritis and rheumatoid arthritis. Pain can be relieved by infiltration of surrounding soft tissues even though injecting specific joints may be difficult.

The *metatarsophalangeal (MTP)joints* are commonly involved in rheumatoid arthritis and overall management will include arch supports and fitted shoes but joint injection under ethyl chloride analgesia may also be helpful. Steroid injections may also play a limited part in the treatment of osteoarthritis and acute or chronic gout. The first MTP joint is best injected tangentially from below the extensor tendon on the medial side using MPAL 1 ml. Other MTP joints will accommodate a smaller volume, perhaps 0.5 ml, and can be injected from the plantar aspect. Steroid injections can also be helpful in a variety of other painful foot disorders, *ligamentous strains* often responding well if steroid is injected into the site of maximum tenderness.

Conclusion

Intra-articular and soft tissue steroid injections relieve symptoms, reduce disability and increase quality of life. They form a valuable part of rheumatology care and are gaining in popularity as their benefits become more widely appreciated. Most of the technical procedures are learnt easily, convenient to perform, inexpensive and carry little risk if done properly. They are well suited to primary care and general medical practice although a number will remain more appropriate to specialist rheumatological practice.

References

1. Dixon AStJ, Graber J. *Local injection therapy in rheumatic diseases. 3rd edn.* Basle: Eular, 1990.
2. Clarke AK, Allard L, Braebrookes B. *Rehabilitation in rheumatology – the team approach.* London: Martin Dunitz, 1987.
3. Doherty M, Hazleman BL, Hutton CW, Maddison PJ, Perry JD. *Rheumatology examination and injection techniques.* London: WB Saunders, 1992.
4. Ching DWT, Petrie JP, Klemp P, Jones JG. Injection therapy of superficial rheumatoid nodules. *Br J Rheumatol* 1992; **31**: 775–8.

12 | Rehabilitation of rheumatic diseases

Anne Chamberlain

Department of Rheumatological Rehabilitation, University of Leeds

Arthritic disorders, despite the many treatments now available, still account for 20% of chronic disability and a loss of some 88 million working days per year. Because of their chronic nature, rehabilitation is essential to the successful management of these conditions. The aims of rehabilitation are to improve the quality of life which might otherwise be disrupted by pain and malfunction, to maximise independence and to restore choice and capability to a level as close as possible to that which existed prior to the onset of disease.

The French equivalent for rehabilitation, *rééducation*, is a reminder that much of the process of rehabilitation is educational, transferring abilities and skills to the patient. It should be seen as a way of enabling rather than simply as a way of doing things to or for patients. As well as being orientated towards realistic and achievable goals, rehabilitation should also be looked upon as a process which is time-limited. This may seem paradoxical when one is dealing with chronic illnesses, such as rheumatic diseases, where it is necessary to retain a clear view of the whole patient over a long period of time. In practice, though, focused care is often necessary at specific intervals because of discrete episodes of joint malfunction.

Because of the many different facets of rehabilitation it is necessarily a process involving a team of skilled workers.[1,2] Although hospital-based by tradition, there is a need for the delivery of such care to take place more in the community. This is possible for a wide range of patients with lesser degrees of handicap, certainly during the more stable phases of illness. Of course, the provision of domiciliary physio- and occupational therapists needs to be sufficient and some of the burden of care will also fall upon social workers and clinical psychologists as well as on the primary healthcare team and informal carers. The model developed for rehabilitation of neurological disease, centred on a team approach in general practice with help from a visiting expert,[3] is easily transferrable to the care of rheumatic diseases.

Impairment, disability and handicap

For optimal management of the rheumatic patient it is helpful to
distinguish between impairment, disability and handicap and to
deal with the problems raised at each of these levels. *Impairment*
indicates a reduction in physical capacity of part of the body, such as
a weak muscle or a stiff joint. Traditional clinical examination
focuses mainly on impairment and this may be necessary or helpful
in assessing muscle function and ranges of joint movement before
and during drug trials or physical treatments. The assessment may
be refined in some cases by the use of various tools. The ability
to grip, which is so important for independent function, can be
measured, perhaps still rather crudely, by using a Douglas bag. A
computer-linked grip-meter, which records maximum grip, endur-
ance and fatiguability, is essential for accurate serial assessments in
clinical trials. The standard clinical examination should also indicate
whether there are other problems which might reduce the chance
or extent of successful rehabilitation, such as marked anaemia or
peripheral neuropathy, heart or lung disease, poor vision or hear-
ing, disturbance of balance or previous stroke.

Disability is the effect of impairment on the patient's ability to
execute specific functions, such as dressing, making a cup of tea or
climbing stairs. Many factors determine disability so it does not
necessarily correlate well with impairment. The same disability may
be produced by a variety of impairments and, conversely, similar
impairments may produce very different disabilities. Disability is
less easily quantified than impairment although it is rather more
relevant to patients' circumstances. Its measurement needs patient
cooperation so factors such as motivation, mood, fatiguability and
attention span may introduce a degree of variability. Physiotherapists are valuable here in their ability to encourage patients
whilst assessing them accurately and safely at the same time.
Depending upon the purpose of the assessment, leg function, as
an example, can be assessed using a dynamometer but whilst it may
be important to assess motor function it is also essential to assess
mobility. Special research equipment can be used to analyse gait
and this has revealed that elderly people prone to falls have great
variability in consecutive step lengths. However, simple methods of
assessment may be quite adequate and for many patients it is
sufficient to measure their ability to climb stairs or to walk a fixed
distance. We do this routinely with children and find that it equates
well with their perceived difficulties.

Handicap is the resultant effect of impairment and disability
on the patient's ability to pursue a preferred lifestyle. For instance,
for a sexually active woman, loss of hip abduction may be a major

handicap and even an indication for orthopaedic surgery. Mobility, which we have just considered at the levels of impairment and disability, can be scored in terms of handicap according to the way in which it allows patients to seek company. Thus, they might be fully mobile or their activities might be limited to the immediate neighbourhood, to the home, to one floor in the home, to one room or even to the chair or bed.

The true degree of handicap may only become apparent when patients attempt to function spontaneously in their usual environment. Identical impairment and disabilities may result in entirely different levels of function at home depending upon personality, expectations, temperament, role, the attitude of the family and the social and physical environment. Patients may be stimulated by the familiarity of their own home and achieve more than seemed possible in hospital. Conversely, activities performed with encouragement in the supervised hospital environment may prove to be unsafe at home or may not be pursued because of an overprotective family.

Assessment systems

There is no universal system of assessment to suit every patient and every purpose but where possible methods should be simple, convenient, reproducible and meaningful. Some are better designed for hospital units and are not always appropriate for outpatient or GP use. Nevertheless, it is important for the rehabilitation team to keep a record of progress and this does require a measurement system of some kind. Ideally, for comparative purposes and to help with communication, methods should be standardised using scales or scores where changes over a period of time reflect real changes in the state of the patient. Ultimately it is important to know whether a patient can function within a given environment so a variety of assessment systems have concentrated on activities of daily living, degrees of dependency, mobility and strength of social support.[4,5]

The *Barthel Index*, a popular rating system for activities of daily living, is simple to apply, has a high inter-observer consistency, is sensitive to change and produces numbers which can be analysed statistically. For each activity, maximum scores varying from 5–15 are given for independence, zero scores for inability and intermediate or zero scores where some help is needed. It assesses feeding, transferring, toilet, continence, dressing, walking and stairs. The maximum possible score of 100, on the modified scale, does not imply normality and changes in score do not always reflect changes in disability. Even so, it is as successful as more complex scoring systems which are more difficult to apply and which take longer to complete.

Various questionnaires are available for assessing rheumatic diseases and these can be filled in by the patient or completed with help using a structured interview. Some are generic and can be applied to a wide range of health problems whereas others are more disease specific. The *Health Assessment Questionnaire* (HAQ) is one of the most widely used for rheumatoid arthritis and the original American version has been modified to make it appropriate for use in the UK.[6] It concentrates on quality of life related to physical function and pain although a modified version includes personal satisfaction ratings. It is simple to complete, it takes less than five minutes and a glance reveals the problem areas to which attention should be directed. It is a great improvement on the old Steinbocker classification which depends on external variables such as employment. The core of the HAQ consists of 20 functions. These include dressing and grooming, rising from a chair or bed, eating, walking, hygiene, reach, grip and outside activities, plus a visual analogue pain scale. Scores for these functions are averaged to create a disability index with a range from 0–3.

The *Nottingham Health Profile* is a generic system for measuring quality of life and it produces reliable and relevant information when used for patients with rheumatoid arthritis and osteoarthritis. It looks at six elements: physical mobility, pain, emotional reactions, energy, sleep and social isolation. There are yes/no responses to a total of 38 items and the positive responses have weighted scores. It has been used as an outcome measure for hip replacement and in therapeutic trials for joint pain.

The *Arthritis Impact Measurement Scales* (AIMS) system has also been widely used for rheumatoid arthritis and it even invites patients to make a priority list for items of care which need improvement. In addition to mobility, physical activity, activities of daily living, dexterity, household activities and pain, it also looks at depression, anxiety and social activities. Its complexity makes it more difficult and time consuming to apply than the HAQ but it continues to be modified and simplified. Another approach, which is highly sensitive to the needs of the individual, is used in the *Goal Attainment Score*. In this very flexible system, the main problems are identified by the patient, the chief carer and the medical staff and specific goals are then set. The success of rehabilitation is then measured by the extent to which these goals are achieved over a period of time.

The assessment of a patient is not really complete without observations on the interactions with family and carers. Rehabilitation may become frustrated when there are unresolved differences in the basic assumptions and goals of those involved in the process. Difficulties arise when patients' expectations are unrealistically high or low or when the family's expectations differ in terms of practical realities from those of the patient or the professional staff. A useful framework for conceptualising types of family and the level of support they are likely to offer may be provided by the *Mutual Support Index*. This defines four family models: the extended family which lives close by and is highly supportive; the modified extended family which lives nearby but offers little support; the nucleated family which lives some distance away and is highly supportive and, finally, the individuated family which lives away and offers little support.

Case histories

Concentrating as it does on function, rehabilitation is rightly concerned with active treatment of the disease itself as well as with its disabling consequences. For example, the 15 year old boy with inflammatory arthritis of the knee, perhaps an early sign of ankylosing spondylitis, needs intensive treatment to the affected joint so that he does not miss vital schooling. In such a case, aspiration of the knee to reduce pain and swelling, injection with steroid to decrease inflammation and encourage compliance, and resting splintage are all helpful in containing the disease process. Intensive physiotherapy, even as an inpatient, then gives the greatest chance of a quick return to his studies.

The teenage girl with aggressive rheumatoid disease illustrates the breadth of the rehabilitation approach and also the need for co-ordination of the many different facets of care. Our patient in question, became ill at the age of 14 with anaemia, polyarthritis and weight loss. The diagnosis of rheumatoid arthritis, uncommon as it is at that age, was delayed whilst it pursued a ferociously aggressive course with rapid loss of cartilage in major weight-bearing joints. Some months after onset of the disease she required a period of hospital treatment to relieve her increasing distress and handicap. A variety of nonsteroidal anti-inflammatory drugs (NSAIDs) were used in high dose during the day to improve symptoms, to reduce joint swelling and to allow intensive physiotherapy. Long-acting NSAIDs were used before bed to improve her quality of sleep and to decrease morning stiffness. Disease-modifying second-line anti-rheumatoid drugs were also started but, because of disappointing results, several were used in sequence over a long period of time.

Rest, graded exercises and hydrotherapy were a fundamental part of both initial and long-term treatments.[7] Splintage was used on her hands and wrists to prevent abnormal and non-functional posture. By day, wrist splints allowed the long flexors to work across stable, more pain free joints and school teachers had to be persuaded that they were useful enough to be worn in class. Resting splints were used during the evening and at night. Night splints were also used for her knees but effective hip splinting was not possible, although night traction helped a little, as did lying prone on the floor whilst watching television. In spite of this level of input, progressive flexion deformities occurred at the hips, resulting in a tiring, poorly functional gait with the Z-deformity of compensatory flexion at the knees.

Over the next ten years she was followed up initially in the regional multidisciplinary juvenile chronic arthritis clinic and later in the adult rheumatology clinic. She continued to receive much physiotherapy and occupational therapy and a comprehensive sequence of NSAIDs and second-line agents. Despite these measures we documented a progressive reduction in the range of movement at various joints. Fortunately, there were welcome improvements in function and restoration of a more normal appearance after expert surgery to her hips, knees and one shoulder.

Surgery

Synovectomy for rheumatoid disease is still regarded as a useful procedure in parts of Europe but it plays a much smaller role in the UK and the USA than it did a decade ago. The initial hope that it would arrest the course of the disease has not been fulfilled and although it can relieve pain, the synovium often soon regenerates. In the hand, tendon synovectomy can prevent tendon rupture but results of joint synovectomy are disappointing and carpometacarpal joints show no benefit after three years. Synovectomised knee joints are no better than unoperated controls after five years but, even so, there is new interest in arthroscopic synovectomy for selected cases.

For joints severely damaged by rheumatoid disease, reconstruction now has an increasing role and multiple joint replacements are not uncommon.[8] Surgery is undertaken to improve function and symptoms but any cosmetic benefit is often appreciated. In the lower limb, hip replacement produces consistently excellent results for pain relief and restoration of function although sometimes there are technical difficulties. In protrusio acetabulae, because of the increased depth of the acetabulum, the forces transmitted through the femoral head are directed unduly medially towards the pelvic cavity rather than through the bone mass of the ilium. During total hip replacement the acetabular cup therefore has to be implanted more laterally to restore the normal line of force up the ilium. This can be achieved by fitting a metal ring to the periphery of the patient's acetabulum or by building up the floor of the acetabulum using bone grafts. Bone can be used from the patient's own femoral head or, for revision surgery, from the iliac crest or a bone bank.

Results of total knee replacement have improved with the use of unlinked surface condylar replacements. With the axial misalignment which occurs in rheumatoid arthritis, collateral ligaments tend to be slack on the convex side and tight on the concave side of the fixed deformity. The shortened ligaments need to be surgically released before implantation of the joint. Central defects in the tibial plateau may need to be filled using bone grafts and lateral defects may also need to be repaired using material from the patient's own femoral condyles screwed into position. The condylar replacements, once implanted, restore the slack collateral ligaments back to their normal length so that they remain taut throughout a full range of flexion and extension and give stability to the new joint.

Ankle arthroplasty is still disappointing and is rarely performed, any component failure causing such large defects in the bone that revision procedures are a major problem. As an alternative, fusion is simple, safe and relieves pain. However, it is not an entirely satisfactory procedure because the rheumatoid foot may also be stiff and deformed at the subtalar and midtarsal levels. In rheumatoid disease the forefoot is more commonly involved than the hindfoot and, although limited surgery to bunions or individual toes may be considered, it is usually better to wait until there is need for resection arthroplasty of the whole forefoot. The best procedure is resection of all the metatarsal heads and sufficient of the metatarsal shafts to correct toe deformities and prevent plantar callus formation. A modification of this procedure is to leave the first metatarsal head and to excise the base of the first proximal phalanx or to implant a silastic joint instead.

Joint replacement surgery in the upper limb is not yet as satisfactory as in the lower limb. At the wrist, arthroplasty has largely been abandoned in favour of arthrodesis which gives strength, stability and pain relief, thus allowing improved hand function. In the hand itself, a silastic trapezio-metacarpal joint can mobilise a thumb fixed

in flexion across the palm. Metacarpo-phalangeal joint replacements are widely used to relieve pain, correct ulnar drift and restore
pinch grip, but grip strength may not improve much because of
poor flexion at the finger joints. There is still a need for satisfactory
interphalangeal joint replacements and in the mean time arthro-
deses may be helpful.

At the elbow, the early hinged arthroplasties often gradually
loosened, causing major problems with revision surgery. The newer,
unlinked surface replacements seem promising, increasing flexion
and rotation without having much effect on active extension. The
outcome is marked pain relief with a welcome improvement in
function.[9] Elbow replacements still carries a high complication rate
with infection and instability in up to 7% and ulnar nerve paresis
which can be permanent in over 6% of cases.

The shoulder joint affected by advanced rheumatoid disease
becomes fixed in adduction and internal rotation and allows very
little elevation. This limitation of movement, especially if combined
with poor flexion at the elbow, makes it difficult for patients to eat,
to place their hands behind their heads, to dress, groom and to
attend to toileting needs. Shoulder joint replacement may produce
a small improvement in elevation and external rotation sufficient to
give a useful increase in function but there may be a tendency to
superior subluxation of the humeral head because of the rotator
cuff which is often ruptured in such patients.

Sequence of surgery

Most patients needing multiple joint surgery elect to have their
lower limbs treated first, perhaps to improve mobility and to relieve
severe pain. Forefoot arthroplasty, if needed, is usually performed
first, otherwise the feet might become unduly traumatised by the
increased activity resulting from more proximal surgery. Hips are
usually replaced before the knees as mobilisation thus proceeds
more smoothly. Bilateral hip or knee replacements may be carried
out at the same operation in fit patients with a reduction in total
duration of hospital stay and without increase in complications.[10]
Alternatively, individual procedures can be performed, separated by
intervals of several weeks or months, preferably with an intervening
period of active rehabilitation at home, rather than during a single
prolonged hospital admission. Any correction to the alignment of
the hindfeet should be performed last.

In the upper limb the wrist is usually stabilised first to improve
pinch grip and hand grasp. Restoration of elbow flexion usually

becomes the next priority, allowing the hand to be brought to the mouth. Shoulder replacement can then be considered so that the hand can be brought to the back of the head and behind the back.

Environment management

Despite the frustrations of mechanical disadvantage, people handicapped by arthritis need to live in harmony with their environment. For this to be possible, the environment may need to be changed or adapted, mediating factors such as equipment aids or appliances may need to be interposed between patient and environment, or the disease state or personal expectations may need to be altered. Patients need to be taught the principles of joint protection from an early stage. The use of a stick or walking aid, taking the car rather than walking long distances, weight reduction and the use of a high chair to reduce the load through joints on rising are all worthwhile measures. Energy conservation reduces fatigue, pain and distress with the prospect of more satisfactory independent living so it should be maximised by detailed examination of life-style. The need to prioritise goals and activities may lead to decisions such as moving from a house to a small flat, or from a country area to be near the amenities of a town.

For many patients with arthritis, problems relating to mobility, seating and bathing can be predicted well in advance so the provision of resources can be made to coincide with the time of first need. A wide range of specific problems may be resolved by an occupational therapist after an assessment of activities of daily living. Standard domestic appliances, such as washing machine, tumble drier, fridge/freezer and food processor, all reduce energy consumption by the user but the single most useful investment for some patients may be a car. Thousands of cleverly designed aids are also available to make life easier and more successful for handicapped people. Some equipment will be obtainable via the domiciliary or hospital occupational therapy service and wheelchairs from the district wheelchair centre.

A visit to a Disabled Living Centre may provide professional advice and demonstrations of other equipment, including driving and domestic modification. The Disabled Living Centre Council, 380/4 Harrow Road, London W9 2HU (tel 071 266 2059) can supply a list of regional centres. Arthritis Care at 18 Stephenson Way, London NW1 2HD (tel 071 916 1500) also gives helpful advice and publishes a regular newsletter. Information on benefits and allowances is often needed and is available from local branches of

DIAL (Disabled Information and Advice Line, DIAL UK, Park Lodge, St Catherine's, Pickhill Road, Balby, Doncaster DN4 8QN, tel 0302 310123).

Conclusion

Rehabilitation is fundamental to the care of patients with rheumatic diseases. It is an enabling process combining the many aspects of disease management, reducing disability and adapting the environment to allow continuing function. Potential for disability exists at every stage of rheumatic diseases so an integrated approach to rehabilitation needs to be used throughout. This calls for a multidisciplinary team where professional skills are used to make accurate assessments, to define realistic goals and to work towards them in an order of priority agreed with the patient.

At times, treatments will take place in hospital. More usually the hospital, with its rheumatology and various outpatient therapy departments, will be regarded as a resource for the patient and community. Increasingly, we can expect to see treatments based nearer the home, usually at the health centre or general practice. Hopefully, therapy will also become more available in the patient's own home.

References

1. Goodwill CJ, Chamberlain MA. *Rehabilitation of the physically disabled adult.* London: Croom Helm, 1988.
2. Clarke AK, Allard L, Braebrookes B. *Rehabilitation in rheumatology – the team approach.* London: Martin Dunitz, 1987.
3. Ward CD, Crates P. Development of a disability team in general practice. *Clin Rehab* 1993; **7**: 157–62.
4. Fitzpatrick R. The measurement of health status and quality of life in rheumatological disorders. *Baillière's Clin Rheumatol* 1993; **7**: 297–317.
5. Barer D. Assessment in rehabilitation. *Rev Gerontol* 1993; **3**: 169–86.
6. Kirwan J, Reeback J. Stanford Health Assessment Questionnaire modified to assess disability in British patients with rheumatoid arthritis. *Br J Rheumatol* 1986; **25**: 206–9.
7. Banwell BF, Gall V, eds. *Physical therapy management of arthritis.* Edinburgh: Churchill Livingstone, 1988.
8. Abernethy PJ. Surgery in rheumatoid arthritis. Problems and prospects. *Proc R Coll Physicians Edinb* 1990; **20**: 52–63.
9. Souter WA. Surgery of the elbow. *Curr Orthop* 1989; **3**: 9–13.
10. Morrey EF, Adams RA, Illstrup DM, Bryan RS. Complications and morbidity associated with bilateral and unilateral total knee artheoplasty. *J Bone Joint Surg Am* 1987; **69**: 484-8.